"It is a common fantasy of psychoanalysts that patients will write about their successful analyses. Generally, such imaginings belong in the realm of analyzable childhood exhibitionism. If this wish were in fact to be granted, it would take the form of Nicola Mendenhall's profound memoir of her 10-year analysis.

Nicola searched without success for a real-life description of how the psychoanalytic process actually unfolds. Her gift is to invite us into that very unfolding. We encounter along with her the oddly asocial relationship that is the psychoanalytic one, as she walks us through the discovery of how it enables her authentic self. We experience through her journey those facets of being human that belong to us all and those that are hers alone. She shares her obstinacy and her vulnerability; her somatizing proclivities and her organic illnesses; her hate for her analyst and her love for her analyst.

Through it all we are right there with her—being confused and frustrated, being enlightened and transformed.

She has provided us what she was looking for—an experience-near reporting of what psychoanalysis is—a human encounter like no other."

Harvey Schwartz, MD
Training and Supervising Analyst
Psychoanalytic Association of New York
Psychoanalytic Center of Philadelphia
Producer IPA Podcast: *Psychoanalysis On & Off the Couch*

"The longest journey is within. Nicky Mendenhall has had the courage not only to travel that searing journey, but with unflinching generous honesty to share it with her readers. Whether they are therapists, clients/patients, both, or those trying to pluck up courage to search for their own freer deep selves, this book offers a guide to the Freudian way of making this crucial journey. Thank you, Nicky!"
- **Trish McBride**, *Exploring the Presence*

"This engaging memoir provides a lucid introduction to Freudian psychoanalysis as the author courageously traces her decade-long journey to uncover repressed fears and mental conflicts."
- **John Broomfield**, *Other Ways of Knowing*

"Fear of the unknown and our courage and strength to face and overcome it seems to be part of every person's life. This memoir helps us to see that while the answer may be simple, the journey to get there is not."

- **Carl Kurtz**, *A Year of Iowa Nature*

"Nicola Mendenhall generously reveals the actual back-and-forth between her therapist and herself during years of Freudian Analysis. From her view, as the patient, Mendenhall shows us why it takes time to change how we think about our lives—which gives us encouragement as we struggle with our own inner journeys.

Dawn Downey, *Searching for My Heart: Essays about Love*

In *Fear, Folly & Freud*, therapist Nicky Mendenhall takes readers into the room and inside her own psyche during her 10-year quest for answers to the issues that plagued her. She offers a disarmingly candid first-person view of why, despite her own training in the field, and despite all external appearances suggesting she had everything one could ask for, she was stuck.

Books on Freudian psychology tend to dwell in the realm of abstract theory, making them at times inaccessible or uninteresting to all but the most tuned in. But between her training and experience as a therapist, her willingness to grow and grapple with self-truths and her endearingly human ability to distill those for others using her life as context, Mendenhall demystifies the territory. We hang in with her struggles, aches and misdirected anger because we care about her. We watch her resist recognizing the roots of her own thought and behavior patterns, realizing how easily we might do the same.

And in the process, maybe we earn some truths about what holds us back in our own pursuits of joy and satisfaction with who we are.

As the book shows, it's never too late to experience that breakthrough sense of true personal freedom that comes with clarity.

- **Rekha Basu,** columnist,
The Des Moines Register

"I have been fascinated with your book, have underlined, starred, put a heart/exclamation point/question mark on almost EVERY page! A lesson we ALL can hear and take in over and over is that we NEVER know what others are going through."

- **Deb Sonner Hubble**—co-writer of
More Than 100 Ways to Learner-Center Literacy

Fear, Folly & Freud

Fear, Folly & Freud

A Psychotherapist in Psychoanalysis

Nicola Mendenhall

Zion Publishing

Copyright © 2020 Nicola Mendenhall

All rights reserved under International and Pan-American Copyright Conventions. No part of this book may be used in any manner without written permission of the author.

All names have been changed except for that of the author, her husband, her three sons, and her four siblings. And all events have been recounted to the best of the author's ability, bearing in mind that the memories we recount are the stories we shape unconsciously in order to justify the way we want to think.

While the author mentions other people in this memoir with whom she has a life, for example—a life with her husband, Wendell, a life as a mother, a life as a grandmother, a life as a psychotherapist, a life as a friend—the only life she focuses on here is her own life with her analyst as guide. The four hours a week Mendenhall spent exploring this inner world changed her, a change she now brings to all her lives.

Glyphs from Vecteezy.com

Cover art by the late Kristi Ylvisaker, Sogndal, Norway

Cover design by Mason Hiatt

ISBN: 978-1-7357958-6-7
Library of Congress Control Number: 2020915056

Zion Publishing
Des Moines, Iowa 50315-1073
www.zionpublishing.org

Printed in the United States of America

I consider the people who have come to therapy as people who have got stuck for lack of alternatives. They come to me in order to increase their possibilities, and it is my function as a therapist to use myself as an instrument to help them.

Salvador Minuchin

Contents

Opening Scene	1
1 Introduction	3
2 Stuck	73
3 The Places I was Stuck	21
4 Just What Is Psychoanalysis?	27
5 What I Wanted = Who I Was	39
6 More Inside Information on Freudian Analysis	53
7 Still Spinning My Wheels	63
8 Stubbornly Still Special	89
9 She Loves Me Most	107
10 My Body Complicates Everything	117
11 All I Ever Wanted Was the Oceanic Feeling	135
12 I Invited Rosanne In	151
13 My World Changes	159
14 Conversations of Transformation	177
15 How Could That Be?	189
16 Preparing to Prepare	203
17 Needing Supplements (Tangible and Intangible)	215

18 I wake up?	231
19 Onward	243
Closing Scene	251
Acknowledgments	255
About the Author	259
Bibliography	261
Recommended Books	263

Opening Scene

"I am curious about the difference between how yesterday's session began and how today's session began." Denae's voice broke into the silence as I settled on the couch.

How fitting that the initial words you read in this memoir describing my experience in Freudian psychoanalysis are words spoken by the psychoanalyst. Words that surprised me, because I had never heard her say them before. Words that implied a question. I remembered how I had started talking as I entered the door the day before. Talking fast.

"Yesterday I was feeling rushed. Today I am not feeling rushed."

"Can you tell me more?"

"When I'm feeling in a hurry, I end up making a presentation."

"Hmmm."

"When I rush, I use words I've always used, often in a know-it-all, above it all manner." I pause. "Now that I think about it, I'm reminded of how Mom made pronouncements, positive or negative, and I went with whatever she said like it was a

fact. It's a whole different story when I don't feel rushed. Then I'm able to take a deep breath and turn inward."

"What does that feel like?"

I move my attention inside. "I see myself wandering around in my interior landscape, a place that has become much more complicated and interesting in the past decade. Before I began analysis, I rarely thought of the farm where I grew up and how I walked gravel roads trying to avoid the gooey mud in the springtime. When I was old enough to drive, I remember being terrified that I would get stuck in the deep. muddy ruts while driving home." I breathe deeply and move into an easy silence. Then a thought, "I always was afraid of getting stuck."

"You're finding psychoanalytical truth."

"Hmmm. Not exactly historical truth but it is the truth of what the present tells me about the past. And the other way around, of course." I adjust the blanket, pulling it partly off my legs while I settle back on the pillow.

There's a comfortable silence before I express the first free association that pops into my mind: "Can we discuss termination?"

"Yes."

1

INTRODUCTION

After proofing this book one last time, I took a deep breath and asked myself: Who in her right mind would spend a decade in therapy and then write a book about it? What sort of person would expose her weaknesses and dysfunctional patterns by writing vignettes detailing her analytic sessions that revealed how stubborn or dense she was? Or how self-absorbed and demanding she could be? Or how much she liked to think of herself as special or above it all? Who would do that?

Writing this memoir has been a profoundly mind-altering, therapeutic process, similar in many ways to the psychoanalytic treatment that prompted it. My first session with a book coach on June 28, 2018, was the beginning of my attempt to describe for others how psychoanalysis changed my life. Since then, with each prod from an editor, with each drop back into the memories of a session, with each revision, I have made new connections and new understandings of the habitual way my mind has worked since childhood.

A few words about classic psychoanalysis:

Freud would have turned 164 years old on May 6, 2020, and his influence is still felt around the world. I have direct knowledge of practitioners in both France and Argentina where his method is still commonly used.

What is the analytical attitude or process that Freud developed? The basic process is this: the analyst listens and gradually develops a clear picture of how the analysand's (the client's) mind works and then, through carefully worded interpretations, reveals what the analyst has learned in a manner that both surprises the analysand and penetrates the analysand's defenses.

When I go back and read from my journals, I'm shocked at how naive and stubborn my responses were to the analyst's well-targeted, incisive interpretations of my motivations. What she said and did brought out the worst in me, eventually shocking me into a more honest self-image.

I suspect you may not like the woman described in the early chapters of this book. While I was writing, I connected with the person I was when in the analyst's office and tried to describe her. As I did, I came to feel irritation and impatience toward her myself.

But I hope you will give that Nicky the benefit of the doubt. Her desire was to grow into what Jennifer Louden would call a "signature theme," which for Nicky was to help others grow toward a more satisfying, fulfilling, and useful life. And, now, Nicky understands that she can only help others if she has first helped herself.

While Nicola was my given name, from the time I was a child my friends and family have always called me Nicky. Through analysis, I have come to realize that clinging to a nickname rather than an adult name was part of my refusal to let go of all the advantages I had as a child. I have had to consciously reclaim Nicola as my name and let "Nicky" indicate familiarity, not childishness.

I hope something about me—the woman who went into analysis as described in this book—will be useful to you. Perhaps the way I saw my life as inadequate and flawed and, at the same time, deprived of something essential, will open your mind to stories you tell yourself about your life. For better or for worse, we all tend to cling to the stories we have created to explain ourselves. And I certainly did.

Perhaps the self-deprecating humor I use occasionally, humor that helps me see the irony of my Big Wants, as my analyst calls them, will give you permission to laugh at yourself and at the myths you have created about your life. Perhaps the openness I tried to practice when recognizing my childhood was idyllic compared to that of many others, will help you refocus your attention from what you didn't have to what you did have.

I sincerely hope that you discover how, by handling the stuck places in my life, I was able to grow into Nicola and then reclaim Nicky as my mature name. I hope these examples can help you identify and move past the ruts or potholes in your own life.

Because I recognize the debt I owe to the many authors who wrote stories of transformation that encouraged me, I hope that my words touch others as I have been touched. I want readers to know that if they are stuck, there is help. They can change. But I also caution them to not be surprised that it takes time and hard work. Discipline and practice. It takes most of a lifetime to grow up.

In fear and humility, I share my story with you, trusting the power of story to uplift and foster change.

Nicola (Nicky) Mendenhall

2

STUCK

If someone ten years ago had told me that a normal, middle-class Midwesterner, who looked, for all intents and purposes, like a thriving American woman in her early 60s, had committed herself to more than a decade of Freudian analysis, I wonder what I would have thought? I suspect I might have wondered (and you may or may not feel the same curiosity) why she would choose to do this? The time? The expense? The energy? But to be perfectly honest, I probably would have been envious of her. I've always been fascinated with people (such as contemplatives or Buddhist practitioners) who commit to long-term inner work. It has been said: If you can change your mind, you can change your life.

I may have continued to ask, despite my coveting her experience, why would she agree to go for analysis week after week, year after year, especially because she was already in her early 60s and had fulfilled a heart's desire and married her high school sweetheart after reuniting with him? And then why, for many years, would she give vague answers when one of the few people who knew she was seeing an analyst would ask her, "How long have you been going?" Or "When will you be through?" Or "What do you talk about?"

While writing this memoir of my experiences in Freudian psychoanalysis, I sometimes asked myself other questions. Why did I begin therapy that fall of 2007? Did it have anything to do with how sick I was with the flu in February of that year, an illness that was difficult to manage? All I can say is that at some level I must have known that I was stuck without a solid sense of self; that something was not satisfying enough with the way I lived my days; that I was not going deep enough into self-understanding to experience the fullness of life.

I knew that I could be funny; but it seemed I no longer felt joy very often. I could be welcoming; but I was always a little fearful and withholding. I could be irritated; but I quickly stamped out any spark of anger, much less rage. I thought of myself as open and accepting; but I caught myself too often sliding into judgmentalism. I was unfailingly sympathetic and helpful when another needed me; but I hoped the person's needs would be temporary.

I might have lived out my life with this level of self-awareness, but for reasons I still cannot fully articulate, I didn't. So over ten years ago, I asked the therapist whose patient I was at the time (all practicing therapists need to have a personal therapist to help ensure their balance and capability) to refer me to someone else, someone who would meet with me more frequently and go deeply into my psyche. He did. But he didn't mention it and I didn't ask, so I didn't know she was a classically trained Freudian psychoanalyst.

Much later, after a decade of intensive Freudian analysis, I struggled to understand what had happened to me. Why did I feel different from the way I felt back in 2007? What had happened that opened for me the possibility of experiencing a wider range of emotions than I could possibly have felt before, moving from annoyance over the needs of others, to fury when I read of injustice in the world; changing from frustration and boredom over the world's problems, to grief over the pain of others; growing from dissatisfaction and confusion over what I needed, to acceptance and delight in what I had. I knew some things were different, but I couldn't explain exactly how those differences played out in ordinary life—and certainly could not explain how they had happened.

The only thing I could do, if someone asked, was to tell them this story. On a damp, raw, autumn evening, I was driving around running errands, and I misjudged the curb on the edge of the road—one of those curbs that are almost non-existent, with only the slightest incline indicating that the concrete ended and the mud of the shoulder began.

I was jerked into alertness when I felt the car bump over the curb—first the front right tire, then the front left. I jerked the steering wheel left and felt the front tire scrape along the edge of the concrete of the road. Quickly I jerked right. Then I felt the flump as one back tire and then the other left the concrete and landed in the muck. I tried again, turning left, trying to return to the road, but I couldn't get up over the edge of the concrete. I gunned the motor, thinking more power would get me there.

That's when I felt the front tires start to spin. I threw the car into reverse. More spin. Forward. Spin. Backward. Spin. I slammed on the brakes. Now what?

All I had to do was call AAA and soon I saw the lights of a tow truck in my rear-view mirror. The driver assessed the situation and saw that going forward was hopeless. So he put a hook on my rear bumper and began pulling me backwards, back and back until I reached the point where I had gone off the road in the first place, the place where he could easily pull my rear tires back onto the concrete, followed by the front tires. "All set, Missy!" he exclaimed. "Just pay better attention when you drive. Stay away from the edge and you should be fine." And off he went.

"It's like that," I would say, "except it took years to get out of the rut I was in, and the only way I would ever be able to move forward in my inner life was, paradoxically, to go back, way back to the experiences that sent me off the road in the first place, to the relationships that had originally fostered my sense of self."

———

I couldn't quite admit how stuck I was when I started what I then called therapy rather than analysis, with what I then called a new therapist rather than an analyst, Denae. I told myself that it would be worth it because, even if it didn't substantially change my life for the better, I would surely learn new methods and skills that I could use in my own therapy practice with clients. I couldn't quite admit, at least not consciously, that I was feeling stuck in important areas of my own life and I needed help in order to understand, in order to find some way of getting unstuck.

If I would have slowed down long enough to realize that I was imagining the therapist would simply pull me out of the muck, like that tow-truck driver who called me "Missy" did, I would have known that my expectations were unrealistic. I was a psychotherapist wise enough to know that I couldn't do this for my clients, and wise enough to know that I was responsible for setting myself on firm ground so I could travel freer and easier on the road of life. But I liked to keep things simple and usually rushed towards closure, so I went into therapy, not recognizing it was Freudian analysis, not recognizing the unconscious rumblings of my inner self.

How naive I was. How childlike in my willingness to want approval and affirmation from this new person. How innocent in my desire to want her to like me and to be her colleague. And then, how like a teenager I was in my resistance to doing everything she asked me to do. I shake my head now, and laugh at all the time I spent during many of those years in analysis both believing that this was the right person and the right kind of treatment for me, and at the same time undercutting her work every step of the way.

I tell you my story with some chagrin, wondering if you, too, feel that restlessness that I felt, if you experience the inability—like my inability—to feel the wide range of emotions available to healthy human adults with a good sense of self; if you have some itch, some undefinable desire, some hope that there can be more to life than what you are experiencing now.

From the beginning of my time with Denae, I was puzzled by her therapeutic method. She never talked! Well, not quite true, but she never talked *with* me. We didn't discuss things. She just sat there and seemed to have no problem with silent stretches. Now, I wonder how I could have been so dense; but it took me an embarrassingly long time to figure out that she was not a therapist like me. She was an analyst. A Freudian analyst.

It took me years to accept her method and to quit trying to either subvert it or convince her to be my colleague. And it took me even longer to understand the difference between what she did and why and how I and others I knew practiced therapy.

Psychoanalysis is over one hundred years old. This psychoanalytic theory of the mind posits that we can trust our ability to face difficulties if we learn to notice and name what rises from beneath the surface of our minds and make choices as to what we want to do with it. The past permeates the present.

Now, more than a decade later and after a massive emotional and financial investment in the process, I would argue with anyone that the process has worked and that my life is better on all fronts.

Toward the end of my analysis, I wished that everyone could experience this transformative process to help them in the areas of their lives where they are stuck. This missionary impulse led naturally to the desire to spread the word by writing.

Once the idea bubbled up to write about my experience in psychoanalysis, I set to work to make it happen. I felt as if I had encountered an "inner necessity"—the words Russian painter Wassily Kandinsky used to describe what motivates the creative process. And what could be a more important (albeit vexing) effort than to begin recreating the process that helped in the recreation of my very self—in spite of the fears that haunted me about exposing myself to both friends and strangers. This missionary inner necessity made me struggle both with doubts that plagued me regarding whether I could describe my analysis accurately and persuasively, and with the insecurities that festered within concerning my lack of training as a writer.

But my biggest fears were that no one would like me if they learned about all my shortcomings, and that they would think—like I sometimes did—that I was stupid. When I began writing, those fears were not as strong as they would have been ten years earlier because I could see and feel changes in myself and in my ways of interacting with my world. But I did sometimes wonder what caused that change and then how it happened. Was it Freudian analysis? Had that huge investment of time and money, not to mention emotional energy, actually borne good fruit?

I have heard that writers write more than they know. Perhaps by recounting for you something of the process and the almost mystical paths my mind took during some of those hours in analysis, I will solve for myself the mystery of what exactly happened and how. And, beyond that, I might shed light on the process in a way that demystifies it for you, perhaps even encouraging you to join me and many others by making an in-depth exploration of your inner life. Through this writing, I also want to move beyond the enthusiasm of a recent convert and into the real world of human behavior and the possibilities for change.

As much as I would have wanted to forget those mortifying insights into myself, those self-absorbed moments of interaction with the analyst, those unfounded assumptions I foolishly made, and the important decisions I based on those assumptions, I am thankful that, right from the beginning, I continued a long habit of journal writing, which started to include documentaiton of what I discovered during analytical sessions. Recollections about my early childhood turned out to be things that were still impacting me, mostly in negative ways. By writing about the discoveries of analysis at the time of the discoveries, I combated my tendencies (unrecognised by me at the beginning) to repress the experiences from my consciousness again.

As you read this memoir describing my experience in Freudian psychoanalysis, you will notice few technical terms. I was meeting with an analyst, Denae, who used common everyday terms as her treatment modality, because she believed that using technical words in the context of analytical treatment would not help in conveying real life. Nevertheless, there were a few terms I needed to understand before I could comprehend what this experience was all about, and you may find a description of those terms useful as well.

The first three terms are *psychoanalysis, analyst,* and *analysand. Psychoanalysis* is mental therapy pioneered by Sigmund Freud. Psychoanalysis is different from *psychotherapy*, which is an umbrella term for therapy practiced according to one of many other psychological theories. Most people working as counselors or therapists fall into the category of psychotherapists. A *psychoanalyst* or *analyst* is a person who provides psychoanalysis, and an *analysand* is the person undergoing analysis. I was an analysand for over a decade.

I reference *free association* frequently, which is a practice of simply letting your mind drift and then naming anything that comes to you when you have taken away all inner editors. Psychoanalysts typically ask their analysands to practice free association as they seek to help the analysands discover what their deep inner drives are.

As I mentioned, Denae used few technical terms, and this mostly let me feel as if I was her peer. Alas, one day she said, "We've talked over the years about *object constancy*.

These words, which she spoke softly, with confidence, caused my throat to ache. I didn't remember what *object constancy* meant.

My voice sounded thin and weak to me as I confessed, "I'm glad you are finally using technical words with me, but I don't know what *object constancy* is."

As always, Denae's statement forced me to deal with feelings. This time, I had to deal with feelings of triumph, because at last she was treating me like the professional I was by using psychoanalytic words, and because I had courage and spoke more honestly than I usually did, admitting my ignorance. But these positive feelings were accompanied by a sick feeling of panic in my stomach. I really did not have any idea what she meant by object constancy and, as someone trained to be a therapist, I felt I should know.

What had we talked about that she was now calling *object constancy*? I was sure those words were never spoken by me. The silence continued and felt uncomfortable.

I had not yet delved into the writings of the famous French psychoanalyst, Andre Green. Waxing poetic about the well-known analytic practice of using silence, Green observed, "silence could be taken so far it was reminiscent of the tomb" (Green, 2005). Lying in silence on the analyst's couch under the analyst's red synthetic blanket (which began to feel like a shroud), I wanted to disappear.

The expensive psychoanalytic minutes continued to accumulate as my feeling of panic escalated. Much to my surprise, Denae spoke: "You know how you say the mother is around the corner and the child doesn't know that the mother is still there?"

"Oh." I breathed a sigh of relief. That's what she meant. I knew about this stage of child development; I just hadn't connected it with the diagnostic name, object constancy.

I remember that incident because it stands out as different. Most of the time she spoke in ordinary language, which left me free to use language in ways that worked for me.

A few other terms crop up but can be figured out by their contexts. The one term I do use often in this book is *unconscious*, which I define in this way:

THE UNCONSCIOUS IS THE HIDDEN, SECRET PART OF OURSELVES THAT WON'T LET US SETTLE.

3

The Places I was Stuck

∞

When I began treatment, I assumed my psychoanalytic sessions with Danae would be more or less like the sessions I conducted as a therapist. I didn't realize that Freudian psychoanalysts worked to unsettle rather than to calm. To that end, Danae created an artificial environment, one where the analyst and analysand met several times a week in an environment where few of the usual social niceties prevailed. Once in this analyst-created environment, I was encouraged to pay attention to things I would usually ignore or think were ridiculous and not worth my time. Also, during that secluded hour, I was encouraged to set aside social norms and express all my inner-feelings, however nasty they may be.

While the word *artificial* in describing the environment may sound negative, I learned that the environment created during analysis is intended be the kind of environment that gives babies and small children a place to thrive—a place where they are supervised but not controlled, encouraged but not forced, questioned but not interrogated, loved but not smothered. In that environment, I could peer into my unconscious and discover which issue I needed to explore. Because my pattern had been to defend against any type of pain, I was shocked by how painful the truth was when I finally faced reality.

The conversations that occurred in sessions were unlike anything I was used to, so afterwards I took time to capture and dissect them so I could learn as much as possible. I started doing research to discover whether what had happened and was happening to me made sense. I thought I was knowledgeable about mental health treatment, having practiced for over thirty years as a therapist, but things that I experienced in that strange environment terrified me, especially the anger I felt.

One late spring day, a few months after beginning my work with Denae, wearing old gray sweatpants, I entered her suite and sat in the waiting room. When she signaled me into her room, I walked briskly in. For some reason, I departed from routine and passed the dark-patterned upholstered chair in need of more stuffing, the chair in which I had always sat, the one that faced the analyst (allowing me to see her eyes), and chose instead to lie on the drab slab of a cot masquerading as a couch where I would try to leave ordinary rules behind. The analyst, now situated above and behind my head, became a sometimes scary, non-visible object. I wasn't sure what was supposed to happen now but knew right away that I had crossed some threshold of trust, where I would be able to be more honest with Denae. And I was proud of myself.

It was several sessions after I traveled to the cot, where in theory I should be better able to free associate (the process whereby the analysand gives voice to everything that comes to mind, with no editing), when I realized I was spending time trying to adjust the pillow so I could be comfortable. The scratchy fabric bothered my neck and lumps poked my head. I punched it this way and that, trying to make it feel comfortable. No use. My eyes blinked rapidly. I wanted to throw the damn pillow across the room. I was pissed. Really pissed. Although I assumed the analyst would give her predictable disapproval, it was not enough to shut me up. I licked my chapped lips, cleared my throat, and voiced my self-righteous opinion in the form of a question, "Do you know that your pillow is hard and scratchy and incredibly uncomfortable?"

My complaint hung in the air for longer than usual, and I waited, tensely, for what I assumed would be her carefully worded interpretation. This interpretation would undoubtedly peg my complaint as an indication of resistance. I began preparing a defensive response. Anyone listening in on my inner dialogue would have heard no hint of shame or uncertainty. I firmly believed I could free associate better if I didn't have to keep adjusting the damn pillow. I knew she was in the wrong for having such a substandard pillow in her office and I felt that I had fulfilled my duty as an analysand when I pointed it out to her. Maybe, I chewed on the idea, I should also inform the Department of Health!

"Do you think analysis is supposed to be comfortable?" she said in an even, no-nonsense tone.

I scrunched up my face and wanted to spit. I bit the loose skin on my chapped bottom lip and swallowed again and again, then forced myself to inhale deeply. I used the pause at the end of the inhalation to silently begin listing the reasons her reply ranked as unsatisfactory. Analysis is by its very nature uncomfortable, so the physical setting shouldn't be! I knew this to be true, otherwise why would I have designed my own therapy office as both comfortable and beautiful. Thinking about my beautiful, safe office brought tears to my eyes. I grabbed some Kleenex and dabbed my eyes and cheeks, then my lips and I saw blood, bright red blood, that must be oozing from the lip I have been chewing. I gave in to angry tears. Then sobs. Meanwhile, Denae sat in silence letting my angry tears turn to sorrowful ones.

While journaling later that evening, nothing in me entertained the slightest possibility that this incident with the pillow would be a harbinger of a major theme I would struggle with for years: the need to be comfortable. No, it's more than that. I demand comfort. But, I rationalized, what's wrong with that? not realizing how every rationalization was like the spin of my tires after I slipped over the curb. It dug me into the muck more deeply and kept me more stuck.

.

4

JUST WHAT IS PSYCHOANALYSIS?

When I sought treatment with a Freudian psychoanalyst, I never dreamed that what I was seeking was a way to find the areas in my life where I was emotionally stuck, to go back to the life situations that prompted that reaction; to feel the feelings I once found ways of avoiding; to release the anger or pain; and then to understand why I had gotten stuck there in the first place. After all that, it would be possible to find another way of moving forward, a way that would lead to adult, mature behavior.

The best way I can describe Freudian analysis, as I mentioned before, is like having someone pull or push you backwards, deep into your childhood, to find the places where you moved off your life's path and began using defenses that protected you from whatever you saw as problematic or dangerous or painful in your ordinary daily life. Erecting defenses is normal. Everyone uses defenses. They only become problematic if, when you are grown and no longer need to protect yourself in that way, you continue to use them, not realizing they will never move you toward mature, loving adult relationships. For instance, an infant cries, and the mother responds by feeding. When the child gets a little older, if words or gestures don't work to satisfy her need because the mother is too busy with other children, she reverts to crying. Before long, crying becomes the automatic tool for the teenager or grownup person to use to get what she wants.

To get unstuck from this knee-jerk defensive way of manipulating others to get what you want, you can use a theory of psychotherapy that gives negative rewards when people behave in these automatic ways and positive rewards when they break a habit and do something more adult. Psychoanalysis, on the other hand, tries to guide the person back to a pre-verbal place of emotion when the habit first began. The task, then, is to express those emotions verbally or through tears. In the example of the girl who learned to cry every time she was at risk of not getting what she wanted, using tears to manipulate people in her world, the emotion she might need to express is anger—raw anger that no one was meeting her needs. Once the anger or rage is released, the person will begin to realize what her behavior is costing her and that she is free to choose a different way, if she has the will to do so. I tell you this so you can read my story through a questioning personal lens, asking how did the narrator of this story react, and how might you have reacted to such efforts by a psychoanalyst? What might work and what would never work for you?

At first, I tried to understand what was happening in terms I knew from my own education as a psychotherapist, but nothing quite made sense. Then I began to research Freudian analytical techniques and then Freud himself.

If I had known that psychoanalysis was a new kind of listening by both parties and that it was different from ordinary psychotherapy in multiple ways, perhaps I would have let down my defenses earlier and made faster progress. Or perhaps I'm using that as my excuse for having made such slow progress for the first years. Change couldn't take so long could it?

Freud didn't discover the unconscious, but he wrote about it and studied it more than anyone else previously had. He used a structural model, as if the parts of the mind were on top of each other and suggested that whatever was in the unconscious level of the mind was there because that thought, image, or feeling was unacceptable to society. Freud supplied the idea of defenses. He wrote that our vulnerable self defends itself by pushing painful things out of reach. Freud believed that it was the painful repressed emotions that caused nervous symptoms (Ragen, 2009). Psychoanalytic treatment aims to coax these banished pieces to return to consciousness and, as Freud said, work them through. Freud believed that anxiety would subside when these pieces were rescued (Dinnage, 1988).

In doing research on Freud and analysis, I was always trying to discover rules that I could use both to govern my behavior in life and to know what was acceptable in session with the analyst. The analyst suggested that there were no hard and fast rules, but that the rules would evolve between us. How could that be? Wasn't there a book somewhere that would outline all the rules? As I look back on those years, I find myself grasping for excuses for why it took me so long—years—to take advantage—full advantage—of the process.

In the Spring of 2009, when I was preparing for my wedding to my high school sweetheart, Wendell, I thought it might be a good time to cut back on my analytical sessions.

It was a Friday morning. Denae and I were in the middle of a slightly awkward session. Her main point (at least that's how it seemed to me) was her accusation (that's what it felt like) that whenever I was upset, I didn't speak up but, instead, shut up.

"When I'm irritable, it means I need time for myself," I said, thinking it was obvious that if I didn't have so many sessions to attend, I would have time for myself, and that not having time for myself was making me irritable.

"You leave when you are irritated—sometimes physically, sometimes emotionally—but you are gone."

"But I need space to integrate what I'm learning," I defended myself.

"The reason to come in frequently is so defenses don't have time to reappear."

I left a silent space in the air while my mind raced. Finally, I asked, "Is my defense denial?"

It sounded like she might be ruminating out loud because the next thing that came out of her mouth was, "I guess I haven't fully understood how intense it must be for you to have a relationship with me."

I decided to ignore her comment. I hadn't assumed she would answer my question, but I didn't totally understand her interpretation, so I wasn't going to speak to it. After a slight pause, she continued: "You are afraid that if Wendell knows how many times a week you are coming, he will look at you like you think people look at your teeth."

That stung. She knew I worried about my crooked front teeth that protruded more than I liked. We've talked about it. Now I wondered, does Wendell notice? I've not worried about that until now as he seems so enchanted with me. I didn't understand what this had to do with anything.

I stubbornly repeated, "But I think it might be a good time to cut back."

What I didn't mention was that part of my desire to cut back was because I was embarrassed. After the wedding, it would be obvious how many sessions I attended a week, so she was correct, Wendell was part of my decision. To be honest, if it was up to me, I probably would have wanted to continue because, even though I was feeling less anxious and could have ended treatment, I still wanted to learn how to balance my emotional responses with self-reflection. And I still thought she could help me. When I really thought about it, I knew I still needed to develop the capacity to tolerate conflict and name it as such. I wanted to continue so I could learn how to stop blowing up and blaming others and learn to keep the struggle within me. These are characteristics I had always wanted but never thought I had, and it felt as if this woman could help me develop them. Plus, I wanted to get to the bottom of my fears and anxieties.

None of this was quite so clear to me at the time because I was operating on autopilot in relationship to my soon to be husband. I had made a mental list of assumptions about what would make him happy and then set about making sure they were all in place.

"You feel as if there is no room for you, no room for your feeling, knowing self. Differences weren't allowed in your growing-up family. You didn't learn that everyone is different," Denae observed.

Rolling my eyes I thought, Boy, she's right about that.

She continued: "I'm not understanding how now is a good time to cut back on our sessions."

Oh damn, was she right again? It probably wasn't a good time to cut back. I wanted my blossoming relationship with Wendell to be as healthy as it could be, which requires time spent together. On the other hand, our relationship would only be as healthy as I was. And I knew I had more work to do.

I could almost imagine her thinking what I had just discovered in my reading about session frequency: "It is common practice in Freudian analysis to have sessions several times a week." She might wonder if I was giving my assumptions about my husband's thoughts more weight than what had been accepted and common practice for decades. Of course, she would never say that—it wasn't her style. But I could imagine the unspoken words. I was smart enough for that. I appreciated that she was tenacious but not authoritarian.

I sat in silence for a few minutes thinking: Maybe I was making assumptions about what Wendell would think. Maybe he would not think that way at all. And maybe, even if he did, that wouldn't mean I should cut back—that would be turning control of my life over to him. I relaxed, thinking about how wrapped up I had gotten in thoughts I was projecting onto Wendell. Wendell doesn't know what I need.

Maybe now was not the time to cut back. Maybe I could learn something from her unyielding belief that, to be successful, we needed four sessions a week. It was only later that night that I realized that she had helped me tune into what I wanted but could not admit. I did want four sessions a week if I was honest with myself. Everything about analysis is complicated. As is everything about relationships. Perhaps she was prescient about my needs.

Before going on, I hope you noticed what happened in that interchange, because it was so typical of our interchanges and always left me confused, until I figured out and understood what she was doing. I would ask what to me was a perfectly legitimate question that could be answered with a yes or a no, and she would take it to a whole other level. She connected my request or question with a pattern in my life that was keeping me stuck. But, since I didn't know what she was doing, for years I was frustrated, until I stopped and asked myself the question, What is she trying to help me figure out about myself? I was always enlightened. An analyst sets this as a goal for her patient—to be able to notice, catch herself, stop, and then question herself, thus breaking the pattern.

According to Freud and psychoanalytic lore, the analyst is to maintain an attitude of neutrality—sometimes called a blank screen on which the analysand's needs and desires can be projected. Freud did not use the words *blank screen*, but continued to develop psychoanalytic practice so it would be non-invasive. The analyst maintains an attitude of observation and inquiry, which are fundamental rules for practicing psychoanalysis. It is widely known that Freud, himself, did not follow these rules. The most favorable theory as to why it is he broke his own rules was so analysts in the future would know what not to do.

I read with both delight and curiosity how Freud and one of his patients, H.D., found release from the pressure of having to always do everything according to his theory and I applied this in my own practice at times. If Freud could twist and bend his own rules, surely I could. H.D. found in Freud's presence warm affection and a very grave philosophy. I noted that H.D. did not seek a cure-all, a heal-all, or a feel-good therapy from Freud, which I think is what I was looking for when I came to analysis. No wonder my analyst had to practice what at times seemed a ruthless, grim, consistency in her loyalty to the fundamental rule: be a blank screen. My neediness made this necessary, though I did not know this for a long time.

―

When I began my own psychoanalytic treatment, I had a vague notion that what I learned might influence my work as a psychotherapist; it wasn't clear to me how true that would be. My analyst's ability to keep her personal life separate from the professional work she practiced initially flummoxed me. I wanted to be her buddy; or at the very least, a trusted, esteemed colleague. While I eventually benefited from her adherence to Freud's idea of the analyst being a blank screen, in reality, most of the time it drove me crazy.

But I knew her style was working for me, so it made sense to me to purchase a couch for my own office. Then I began sitting at an angle where my clients couldn't see me, after, of course, a detailed explanation of what benefits they would gain from lying down and facing the other way. I told clients how I was obtaining psychoanalytic supervision and studying the literature. This change in how I practiced was particularly difficult for one of my long-term clients who was used to being able to see my support and responsiveness. For the most part, even she was able to discern how the new arrangement was working to her advantage. Granted, occasionally she would twist her neck around so she could see me after she said something outrageous, but usually she was a model psychoanalytic patient.

One day after she described a multitude of life issues (a job change she didn't want, a parent's illness that probably wouldn't improve, a delinquent daughter in danger), she began to weep. She asked me in a little-girl voice whether I thought she was handling these issues well.

Her question startled me, and I was glad she couldn't see me because she would have seen my wide-open eyes and look of shock. She had worked with me long enough to know that my likely answer would be to direct the question back at her and help her explore how she felt she was doing. I knew this from my own experience: when I came to a determination about myself regarding my performance rather than hearing praise from someone else, it was much more powerful and lasting than anything the analyst could have said. As my face softened and our breathing slowed, my intuition kicked in and I knew that there was something about the squeak in her voice I needed to pay attention to. It was clear to me that she needed a different answer. She needed a compassionate response.

As she stood, she turned to me, a haunted look on her face, a look that cried out for affirmation. So, I nodded my head and murmured to her that, yes, she was doing quite well. She nodded, almost imperceptibly, and began getting ready to enter into the cold vast outdoors. I nodded back. That was all she needed.

And for me, what I needed was to begin to trust my own instincts for when to stick to a strict adherence to Freud's principles and when to trust my own.

5

WHAT I WANTED = WHO I WAS

From the time I was a young woman, studying clinical social work and psychology and practicing as a therapist, I had a therapist of my own, as is the common practice for therapists. Late in my career, I began feeling the need to find someone new, someone more demanding. My desire for deep personal transformation, always present in my psyche, began escalating while reading accounts of other women's personal transitions.

A *Walk on the Beach* (Anderson, 2004) described the author Joan Anderson's summer away from her husband, pursuing her own personal growth (a situation that mirrored a dream I had had for years). Joan befriended another Joan, an elderly woman who became a trusted mentor. Intimate walks on the beach with a trusted older woman appealed to me after nearly a decade of dating unsuitable, unavailable men. As Joan's story unfolded, it became clear that the elderly Joan was tending her husband, the famous psychologist, Erik Erikson. It felt like I knew her because I knew of him from my studies in social work. Both Joans inspired me with their deep need for personal space, contact with the arts, and familiarity with the unconscious. Their stories whetted my appetite for my own personal work.

Leaving the Saints (Beck, 2005), by Martha Beck, was a gift from my sister Nina, who said she enjoyed reading the book and, in a way only Nina can, strongly suggested I read it. Since the book described Beck's departure from The Church of Jesus Christ of Latter-Day Saints, it triggered issues around my own connection to institutional Christianity, in which I had been raised and which I saw from the inside during my first marriage to a church administrator. I was eager to read her experience. Another draw for me was that I had lived and worked in Utah at the time of my first marriage, so I knew the power of the LDS church. Bowled over by how Beck explored her religion and found her spirituality, I kept reading. For almost a decade, I struggled with the issue of whether the United Methodist church would continue to be part of my life. Maybe this new therapy would bring me clarity on my connection to the church and focus my spiritual yearnings, as Beck had focused hers.

The book *Eat, Pray, Love* (Gilbert, 2006), popular enough to be on the best seller lists, appealed to me primarily because India—a country I love and had visited on two occasions—was one of the three countries Gilbert wrote about (Gilbert, 2006). Each time I visited India, my eyes had been opened a little more. The colorful Indian culture made my surroundings in the U.S. appear bland, though upon returning home, I always vowed never to return. I did not want to again put myself through viewing the human pain and suffering I saw on the streets and, also, the stress on my body. Listening to a deeper desire than comfort, I returned two more times in the next few years. Something about India appealed to me and frightened me—not unlike psychoanalysis, I thought with a grimace. Gilbert visited an ashram while in India, so her experience was different from mine. Regardless of these differences, I still felt I was living vicariously through her when I read of her adventures. The new perspectives that she claimed to have acquired were tantalizing to me. Maybe, I thought, my new adventure into in-depth therapy would give me some of the courage and insight Gilbert exhibited.

These three books, in addition to scores of others, described how living into the paradox of certainty and surrender, being open to adventure, learning that you cannot do it on your own, and undergoing intense therapy were able to work toward personal transformation. This was what I longed for. Transformation beckoned me. Would this new therapy change me as much as each of these women were changed? Would my training as a therapist help or hurt my chances?

⁂

I assumed, without knowing I was assuming, that I would have an intimate relationship with this new therapist, that she would recognize me as a colleague, that she would treat me as someone special—perhaps even offering me friendship. I expected that, at the least, she would share her thoughts and insights about me as we went along, insights that would help me know her, even as she was getting to know me.

To consciously have known that I had these assumptions would have reminded me of difficulties I encountered with my clients who wanted to cross the boundaries I established, clients who didn't know how to see me strictly as their therapist but wanted to be friends. But I didn't put these two things together. These books, telling the stories of other women's transformations, raised the bar of my expectations and stoked desire in me. I wanted to be changed and, as a part of that change, and as a way of professionally justifying the time and expense, I wanted to learn new strategies for working with my difficult clients, clients who had issues similar to mine.

By the time I walked across the parking lot for my first appointment with Denae, my underarms were beginning to sweat. Did I forget to put on deodorant? I must be feeling minor anxiety at the thought of meeting this new person. But when I drove down the street, a sense of familiar ease swept over me. A memory became more conscious with every breath. My internship supervisor, a woman who generously supported me, lived on this street (though I'm not sure how I knew this fact because I never visited her). How strange that I had thought about her now. How delightful that my mind gave me what I needed to feel calmer.

As I approached the inconspicuous threshold that would lead to my new therapist, all the healers I had worked with in the past floated through my mind. The biofeedback expert who was impressed with how fast I caught on and complemented me so lavishly that I didn't trust her. The massage therapist who lectured me on the shoes I wore. The acupuncturist who tested me for food allergies using a special method that looked a lot like magical thinking. The psychic who told me that my partner wasn't ready yet but that he would be coming. The spiritual director who gave me books to read. My time with each of them boosted my self-esteem, gave me something new to think about and disappointed me. As I bade each of them farewell, I knew I wasn't finished with myself.

⁂

I take a deep breath and open the door to the new therapist's suite on the second floor. Soft music floats in the air. No artificial aroma used to mask the old building smell, thank heaven. Draped tweedy looking throws, comfy chairs, muted light and dark colors. No one visible. I notice a closed door on the left-hand side of the room and assume it's where she is. I feel a twinge of disappointment.

When new clients come to my office, I try to greet them. I know that, at least for most people, the decision to begin therapy is difficult. Here in this unfamiliar suite, I stand in the middle of the room. Just breathe, I tell myself. Give her the benefit of the doubt. Assume she is with someone else and having a hard time ending the session. Probably doornob therapy, I reason—

the name we give for the crises that are brought up in the last minutes of a session.

I begin to fill out an intake form clipped to a clipboard strategically placed on an end table. While I am filling it out, I wonder how much of myself to reveal. I am a seasoned psychotherapist and I don't know her. How detailed should I be?

The door opens and she appears. She walks like my osteopath advised me to walk, her feet slightly pointed out, giving the impression that she glides. She looks me in the eye and smiles briefly.

"Call me Denae," she says as she takes my forms, hands me a business card, and leads me into the consultation room.

I look at her card. I must have a question on my face because she responds as if she is answering a question:

"It's pronounced Den-ae. My mother wanted a name that would be easy to pronounce but many people have trouble with it."

It will be years before I realize the rarity of that moment. I merely nod, she nods, and I nod back, tucking that little tidbit away and thinking, well, we are off to a good start. She has revealed something of herself to me. Now it's my turn.

There was no way I could have known that this would be one of the few things about herself she would ever tell me.

As we continue to move into the slightly larger consultation room on the right, I notice several places where she might sit and wonder where she wants me to sit. When she fails to give any direction, I choose a seat where I will not have to look into the light, as brightness makes it difficult for my eyes to see—not a big problem here, since heavy drapes on the windows block the view and the sunlight.

She sits down across from me, looks at me, but doesn't move her mouth to speak. She sits there. If she had been on the floor cross-legged, sitting on a meditation cushion, I would have thought she was settling in for a long meditation session.

After extracting a Kleenex from my sleeve (mostly for something to do as my nose is not really in need of immediate attention), I raise the tissue to my nose and blow softly. While internally debating how to dispose of the lightly soiled Kleenex after this *faux* nasal emergency, I remember my dad's observation that I always left a trail of Kleenex behind like breadcrumbs. I decide to save the Kleenex in my purse that I have placed carefully on the floor by my feet. I purposefully open the purse, the zipper making an alarmingly loud noise in the silent room, and peek briefly into the interior as if I am looking for something. Remembering that I am on a mission to deposit the Kleenex, I do so and look up to see what she is doing. She is still there, just sitting. I feel uneasy. Isn't she going to begin the session? I wait a few moments.

Finally, unable to endure another minute of tension, I speak. "I don't know how much you know about me, but I am a licensed clinical social worker and a licensed marriage and family therapist. I've had my own solo practice for about twenty years."

I look more closely at her, trying to determine what she is thinking. Is she impressed? Her expression remains neutral. I can't tell. I begin to feel sweaty again and quickly return to my introduction. "I am a mother of three grown sons, a grandmother of two girls and two boys, a sister to four siblings. I was an only child for six years and then a sister arrived, Nina."

I pause, waiting for her to say, "How did that change things?" Something I would have asked a client. But she remains silent. "Then, the next year they get their son, Nolan. Three years later, another sister was born, Nan. And finally, the last sister was born, Nyla. I was fifteen by that time, and not home much." Again, I pause, wondering if she will pick up on that. Her face remains enigmatic. "I have lived alone since my divorce ten years ago from the father of my children. Our marriage lasted for over thirty-three years, with the first fifteen years being relatively happy." Again, no comment. No "How did that feel?" No "Tell me more about that."

I go on, and the more I discuss my life, focusing on the positive aspects of what I possess and have accomplished, the more confidence I begin to feel. This is kind of fun after all. But as quickly as that thought crosses my mind, irritation arises, and I wonder, Why am I here? Why had I made this appointment? I have a lot going for me! I don't need this.

And beyond that, Why is she behaving this way? She's getting on my nerves. I pick up my purse again and pull out the Kleenex. This time I don't even bother to blow my nose but place the Kleenex in my sleeve where it belongs and drop the open purse loudly on the floor. I recall, while driving to the session, worrying there might be too much material to cram into a mere fifty-minute hour. I push my sleeve up, hoping to see my watch. The Kleenex threatens to fall out, but I push it back swiftly and look at the time. I hope she is not looking. I am surprised so few minutes have passed. When I eye my watch, I have more time left than I thought. What else does she need to know about me?

Her lack of responsiveness begins to trouble me and make me anxious. She looks perfectly calm and relaxed in her chair, holding her paper and pen, and taking notes occasionally. When I look at her, she looks back, expectantly. She seems ready to wait indefinitely.

This is not going the way I thought it would. Or should.

Denae (What a weird name, I think), doesn't seem impressed with my life, like most people are when I introduce myself. Not only is she not speaking to me, I don't see any non-verbal reassurances either, no head-nodding or murmurs of encouragement. I look around the room and my eyes rest on the large painting on the wall adjacent to me, directly above a cot-like couch with a slanted pillow. I wonder if people really lie down there. The picture is of a woman staring off into space and reinforces my question of why I am there. What is she looking at?

But, then I remember the problems I encountered finding a therapist. I know so many therapists in town after having lived here so many years that it is difficult to find a therapist I don't know either professionally or socially, one whom I would feel comfortable seeing for treatment.

I realize suddenly how much I want this to work. It has been exciting to anticipate the possibilities of forging a new relationship and learning more about myself. I yearn for the type of intimacy that I read Joan Anderson found with Joan Erikson walking on the beach. The silence continues. I am becoming increasingly uncomfortable.

Then, tears come to my eyes as I hesitantly say, "I have a lot of fears."

I expect her to ask me what fears I am referring to but, instead, my revelation is met with more silence. Silence that is thick and impenetrable. It doesn't appear she is going to ask me what fears I am talking about, so she must be waiting for me to tell her.

I begin with the easiest to admit. "I don't like driving, because I can't see very well and have no sense of direction, so I tend to get lost. Once I even ran off the road. Every time I set out by myself I feel a rush of fear."

I want her to say something like, "Well, that sounds like a reasonable fear." But, still, no response.

At this juncture, it would have been difficult for me to articulate the fact that reassurance and comfort were not always the most compassionate response for a therapist to make, because I had not yet learned this bit of wisdom. I usually erred on the side of positive mothering with my children and encouraging words with my clients.

I desperately want to receive reassurance and comfort from her right now.

The silence deepens.

Finally, I find courage to share more of my fears:

"I really am afraid of getting lost, plus I am afraid of water."

No response.

I throw in a very female fear that feels shameful when I admit it, but it was screamingly true, so I don't dare leave it out.

"I am terrified of mice."

The silence feels awkward. Could it be important? She seems to know what she is doing but I sure don't.

At last, with only a few minutes left, she offers a few words:

"Do you want to reschedule?"

I'm astonished. Did I or didn't I? She operates so differently from what I am used to. I have no clue what she is doing or if it will do any good. And yet, I am intrigued by this mysterious method that seems so simple on the surface—at least for the analyst. All you have to do is sit there. But it couldn't be that simple, could it?

I open my date book. We schedule two sessions for the next week. I don't know what I am getting myself into, but I am resolute that I want to continue, at least until I understand who she is and what she is doing.

And only now, as I reread what I have written, do I grasp the irony of being more interested in understanding the therapist than in what she could do for me. At the time, I had no clue that anything was odd about going to therapy to figure out the therapist rather than figuring out yourself.

6

MORE INSIDE INFORMATION ON FREUDIAN ANALYSIS

∽

Four years later, while lying on the couch (with my knees tented to the ceiling, so the blanket could be doubled up for warmth and cover my calves), my mind jumped to another time I was worried about keeping my legs warm. I began to tell Denae about the time my Tai Chi teacher asked if our class wanted to practice in the courtyard. I turned up my nose in disgust. I didn't want to go outside. It was windy. I saw lilacs in bloom and figured they might bother my sinuses. It was chilly outside; I might catch cold. I might get a headache from the wind. Why couldn't she just let things stay as they were? It was perfectly nice inside. I looked down at my sandals and then out at the irregular steppingstones that made the pathway and pictured twisting my ankle.

All the people there, including the teacher, looked as if they wanted to go outside but must have sensed that I did not because suddenly the teacher said we would stay in. I breathed in deeply and mused that I was either powerful or narcissistic for believing I had affected the outcome. Feeling victorious, nevertheless, because I had gotten my way, I settled into practice. It was short-lived. A chill ran down my spine as the sun peeked out from behind the clouds. The room with its beige curtains and dirty carpet started to feel sterile and ugly. It was chilly with the stupid air conditioning running full blast. I moved my arms in the circular movements I loved and peered outside again at the beauty.

Opening my arms wide, I said dramatically, "Let's go outside!" Everyone cheered and clapped.

"Why do you think initially you didn't want to go outside?" Denae interrupted the end of my story before I could tell her how wonderful it had turned out to be outside.

Immediately upon hearing her question, I pictured walking down the gravel road towards my grandparent's house, leaving my mother behind at home, believing that she did not like the outdoors. I assumed that Mom wanted me to be inside with her, but I wanted to be outside.

I had processed differences between me and my mother with the analyst. Mom wanted me in with her while I wanted to be outside. This was confusing. So, the fact that I did not want to go outside for Tai Chi puzzled me, because it was the opposite of what I would have preferred as a child.

But suddenly I had a flash insight: "Maybe Mom wanted me to be outside so she could have time to herself inside, but I wanted to be inside because I assumed she needed me," I said with a hesitant voice to the analyst. This was a totally new thought. I had always thought the reason I did not like to be outside as an adult was that I had given up the joy of the outdoors to help my mom inside. But, perhaps I had needed to think that. Maybe she didn't need me as much as I needed to be needed.

"Where do you think that flash came from?" the analyst asked me, almost in a whisper.

"I think it was from my unconscious," I said while still feeling confused about the challenging new thoughts I had uncovered. I wanted things to be simpler. It was not until later that I was able to comprehend my unconscious was attempting to help me gain a clearer picture of my mother. My mother was not one-dimensional or consistent. And, I was to learn, neither was Freud.

An amazing thing happens when you have a subject on your mind. You begin seeing it everywhere. This certainly was the case when I became open to learning about Sigmund Freud. Nearly every book that contained an index in my collection had at least one—often many—page numbers after the words *Freud, Sigmund*. Books without indexes surprised me by mentioning Freud on the first line of their introductions.

For example, in *Going on Being* (Epstein, 2001), Mark Epstein introduced what he said was an obscure story about one of Freud's personal conversations. Although I had been skeptical of Epstein's promise of obscurity, the anecdote was one I had not read, but found very moving.

In this story, Freud was conversing with Ludwig Binswanger, a Swiss psychiatrist. Binswanger believed there was something missing in Freud's approach to therapy and raised the problem he named, the *paralysis of analysis*, by asking Freud a question: "Might there not be a deficiency of spirit?"

Much to his amazement, Freud readily agreed: "Yes, spirit is everything."

Binswanger was surprised at this answer and thought Freud must have misunderstood his meaning of *spirit*, thinking perhaps Freud thought he meant *intelligence.* But Freud continued: "Mankind has always known that it possesses spirit. I had to show that there are also instincts" (Epstein, 2001).

Freud felt strongly that Judeo-Christian culture was not enough to manage the antisocial proclivities of humans. He thought the intellectual elite would be open to a universal science-religion or a veritable religio-mystical psychology. Freud made sure psychoanalysis had a fundamental tenet that would clearly state his belief that there was not a deeper, religious layer to the unconscious. He believed the road to healing opened if the analyst could interpret psychoanalytically the insights from the unconscious.

As I began to immerse myself in the psychoanalytic process, the mysterious content of my unconscious continued to reveal itself to me. I would find myself in an experience that was teaching me what I needed to learn while teaching me something that my unconscious had kept secret.

One day, while sitting in a coffee shop, I superimposed two parts of my life (the self that was a therapist and the self that was receiving therapy) and created a fantasy about the strangers I saw across the coffee shop—two people who, I imagined, possessed rich, full, inner lives, who draped themselves on the well-worn leather couches, thought deep thoughts, and had meaningful conversations. Perhaps this meant that I wanted a therapeutic relationship with that kind of ease.

Or, maybe my desire to lie down on the therapist's couch was based on vague fantasies fueled by portrayal of psychoanalysis in the movies. I might not have been so eager to occupy the couch had I known that Freud, in his 1913 paper:

> "On Beginning the Treatment," listed strict guidelines for his patients who were on his couch. Psychoanalyst Theodore Jacobs writes: "Freud made it clear that the patient needed to be instructed, not only to say everything that came to mind, but, quite explicitly, to avoid the temptation to withhold any thoughts, no matter how distressing or embarrassing" (Seulin, 2012).

Free association, a key process in psychoanalysis, requires mentioning everything that comes to mind without editing out any content. This was not an easy thing to do. This terrified me—what if I insulted my analyst? What if I said something I did not want her to know? So, rather than lie on the couch and let my mind go in free association, I reported on my preplanned associations which became more and more difficult to formulate as time went on. Some days I didn't have a clue what I wanted to talk about.

During all this time, I kept mining the literature for information about this kind of analysis. In *Freud and Beyond*, I spied a clue as to what free association was all about: "By encouraging the patient to report on all fleeting thoughts, the analyst hopes to get the patient to bypass the normal selection process that screens out conflictual content" (Mitchell S. A., 1995).

Aha! Now I knew what she was looking for: Conflicts! Any kind of inner dissonance. The kinds of things that keep you awake at night. Things that cause you to wrap yourself in self-righteousness; slide into despair; become filled with fear, anger or confusion. Does this mean I am supposed to talk about all that? I didn't believe it would be good for me to stir up all those old feelings. So I didn't for many years.

I kept learning more and more about psychoanalysis. I couldn't seem to stop reading and collecting quotes like this: "In the strictest applications of the classical method, the analyst does not ask questions, and within the logic of the classical model, this is as it should be" (Mitchell S. A., 2016). As you read this memoir, note how few questions Denae asked.

The neutrality and nondirectedness of the classical Freudian method, I discovered, protected the patient's autonomy and guaranteed that the deepest levels of the patient's conflicts would be accessed. The analyst tries to be scrupulous when it comes to not influencing the patient.

However, in reality, often while on the couch, I return to my old habit of obsessing about what the other (in this case Denae) is thinking about me. I think she likes me. But … sometimes I am not so sure. We keep going over the same things. It's true that each time I feel a little different. But doesn't she get tired of me?

As much as I hate to admit it, as my analysis went along, I withheld my thoughts more times than I can count. I had limits to the personal information I was willing to share with the analyst. For instance, for a long time, I refused to share with Denae any information about sex with my husband. Finally, I discovered that, the more I trusted and expressed my free associations, the more I learned and the more clearly I saw my thoughts, my actions, and my interactions. I also realized what should have been obvious to me as a therapist: withholding my thoughts was a waste of time and of money.

I was relieved to read that, when in analysis, one is constantly in the throes of not knowing. And I, eventually, learned that being in the throes of not knowing was where I needed to be. But, in the meantime, I was determined to figure it out. I needed this to make sense.

7

STILL SPINNING MY WHEELS

I remember reading Michael Sledge's memoir where he confessed he could not picture himself lying on a psychiatrist's couch without laughing out loud at the sheer melodrama of it. I related. I wanted analysis and yet I continued to resist. A journal entry, written in early September 2007, about a month before my first session, asserted that my first appointment with the new therapist was scheduled but I did not mention anything about psychoanalysis.

In a different journal, in an entry for September 27, 2007, I wrote: "I can't believe that I have an appointment on Monday to see a counselor that does psychoanalytic work." I do not know how I learned she practiced psychoanalysis. I obviously was ambivalent towards change. I imagine I went because the force of my unconscious desire to stop spinning my wheels, to move forward, was increasing. Little did I know that before I could go forward, I had to go back, way back to my childhood, to the place I had gotten off track.

What I want you to know by telling you my story is how difficult it is to make deep changes in your behavior and how many mental games you play to avoid every painful awareness. I also want you to know that when things in your life become difficult, that, too, is part of the process. It took me years to realize that I had to stay with the pain in order to get through it. This chapter may be a challenge for you to stick with because, as the title indicates, I spent years spinning my wheels (metaphorically speaking). I am going to share with you embarrassing things about my process and the mistakes I made, because I hope knowing (what I came to think of as my folly) will be helpful as you continue your own process. So slow down and pay attention to ways your own unconscious will try to make itself known to you. I can guarantee it will. The hard part is noticing and then paying attention and then acting on it. I know, I know, that is more than one hard part.

I did not consciously know I was spinning my wheels before I started psychoanalysis. I always was investigating new ways of being, though in reality, I usually ended up discarding new theories and justifying my old ways of thinking and feeling because the old ways were so comfortable and for the most part worked pretty well. I will share with you what I wish I had been able to hear during those early years of analysis. There were three patterned ways of thinking, or you might call them mindsets, that I was too stubborn to even be conscious of, let alone release.

The first was my desire—my need—to be my analyst's colleague. But rather than admit that to myself or share these feelings with her, I silently argued with her and second-guessed her methods. Concealing my reactive behavior and ways of thinking made it almost impossible for me to free-associate, because I was always thinking to myself that I could not reveal this or that thought because it was too immature. I wanted her to see me as a sophisticated professional who knew most everything she knew. I wanted her to see me as her peer.

Are you ready for an embarrassing part? Do you ever have fantasies? I concocted a fantasy which gave me great pleasure every time I avoided reality and indulged in it: The initial scene features the two of us professionals (Denae and me) meeting at the local coffee shop, huddling over hot drinks (Jasmine green tea for me), laughing with our heads tipped towards one another, marveling together about a controversial book which we both read in which the author experimented using Freud's technique on psychopaths. We are amazed at the insightfulness, the wisdom, the sheer genius of the author's words in the book's foreword. He proclaims that practitioners of psychoanalysis are the "objects of veneration and fear"; and are "on their way to elevation as priests" (Lindner, 1982). We wink at each other with pleasure when we see the word priest used to describe us, because we share spiritual inclinations.

But we laugh the loudest—louder than the coffee grinders in the background and so loud other patrons swivel their heads around to see us—in our frank admiration for the author's cleverness describing those who have lain on couches as "the saved, the latter-day community of saints whose canceled checks comprise a passport to heavens denied those less favored by fortune."

This rendition of our dear clients is almost too hilarious for us to bear, though at some level we hope it is true. We order another round of beverages and add a biscotti to split. Our discussion is fervent. We wonder aloud if the author has gone too far when he calls us a "kind of devil's disciple who uses arcane and mystic means to secure transformation of character" (Lindner, 1982).

We each have clients waiting back at our offices, so we draw the banter to a close. We shake hands, then briefly embrace as we agree whole-heartedly with the author's last paragraph that points out the analyst's own person is his or her only tool. I imagine my analyst later telling a colleague about her new friend and peer—me.

It took me a long time to recognize the way I used this particular fantasy as a way to affirm my professional status—in fact, raise my status—by being a companion of my analyst. I had an instinct to set this fantasy in a coffee shop, even though I didn't yet know how much coffee shops—a place where peers gather—had come to be a cultural metaphor for intimacy, knowledge, and understanding.

Years later, in the process of editing this memoir, I reread what I had written about the coffee shop. A rush of shame came over me and I was tempted to delete it. It embarrasses me, even now, how I let my mind concoct coffee house fantasies. What an indication of what I later learned (through analysis) was my need to be special. How could I ever get unstuck from that need to be special when I couldn't even recognize it in its most blatant form?

I would not have admitted this to Denae. Admitting to my fantasy would be tantamount to confessing that I was stuck in the muck of my need to be special, to be #1. In addition, my fantasies usually contained tidbits about Freud or about analysis that I had been discovering in my reading of books about Freud, books that I mistakenly believed were off-limits for me during analysis. Later I realized that because she did not want to recommend a book to me didn't necessarily mean she didn't want me to read at all.

This brings up the second area in which I was stuck in old thinking. My immersion in psychoanalytic literature arose, at least in part, from my unrecognized wish to be someone people looked up to intellectually. This, of course, also put me on an equal level with Denae as her full-fledged colleague. But it was more than that.

Surrounding myself with books had always eased my anxiety that I did not know enough, that I was not a brain—as the smartest kids in the class were called, as Wendell was called. I realized in retrospect that I expected to be smart without having to study. I was gobsmacked when Wendell told me how much he studied in high school and college and how, during the four years he was in college, he did not attend one college football game but instead went to the library to study and read.

As a girl, I had used reading (something my Mother liked to do herself) to escape from being her little helper. I loved a good story about how others dealt with their lives and relationships. All my life, because of curiosity and sometimes the need to escape, I have loved to read.

But one day while investigating psychoanalysis, I happened upon a chapter describing psychotic breakdowns. I skimmed those pages, freaking out when I imagined myself having a psychotic break and being hospitalized. Or, I envisioned kicking the analyst, behavior I read could happen if I had a breakdown during a session. Could these things happen to me? Apparently. They happened to others.

I briefly considered putting my books away for the duration of my analysis, but I couldn't. The habit was too ingrained. The need for escape too great. The emotional pothole too deep. I kept reading and satisfied myself that such a breakdown would not happen to me. I was, after all, special.

The third way I was stuck was my knee-jerk ability to rationalize or justify anything. I used my brain to gather information and then to find ways of thinking about things that helped me feel good about myself. For instance, when I decided to keep reading books, I rationalized that it would benefit me to know more about the theory behind psychoanalysis. I recognize now that this response was another indication of how I was stuck in the habit of rationalization or justifying everything I wanted to do or any way I wanted to think. So, I continued to undercut Denae's efforts to help me session after session, year after year. I sheepishly remember a particularly obvious example—though not at all obvious to me at the time.

One Tuesday, I broke an unconscious rule of arriving for sessions no earlier than a minute before the scheduled session time and arrived a good five minutes early. As I walked into the building, I contemplated why it had always felt so important not to be early but dismissed the question quickly. Sometimes it was just too much work to think psychoanalytically. It then flashed through my mind that even Freud said sometimes a cigar is just a cigar. I should look that up, I thought; I wonder if he really said that?

I sat down in the waiting room and thought briefly about picking up one of her magazines, all of which were several years old. I decided against it. I looked around. Nothing ever changed in this waiting room, I murmured to myself. The wooden credenza with multiple drawers, which tempted me to peek inside, sat motionless. But wait, were the lamps new? Most things in this office used straight lines but these were pleasingly rotund. They were made from shiny, earthy ceramic! They must be new!

I'll ask her, I thought. She will appreciate my sharp eye for changes. She couldn't get two new lamps without my noticing! So, I began the session by asking, "Are the lamps in the waiting room new?"

"Tell me more," she replied.

My response (inwardly) was to chide myself for even asking. I should have known after years in analysis that she wouldn't answer a straight question. But I couldn't help but persevere, "I like the lamps and think they must be new because I don't remember seeing them before."

"What do you imagine?" she countered.

My whole entire inner being shrieked: This is ridiculous! Why won't she just tell me? She doesn't need to keep treating me like a patient. Why doesn't she just tell me why she's not telling me, and I will understand, and we can get to the real work of analysis.

My mental temper tantrums used great energy to get nowhere.

But this was just the beginning.

As part of Denae's efforts to delve into what I was not provided during my childhood, she kept nudging me toward revealing more and more about my relationship with my parents. My rational mind would say to anyone: my mother was my most important parent, the one

I loved and counted on, the one who gave me all I needed to grow up. But thoughts of my father kept interrupting my reveries. For instance, he was present each time I used his favorite word *ridiculous*. I knew my dad would have thought going to analysis was *ridiculous*, a term he used for anything he didn't understand or was fearful of. And yet, it was ironic that I felt him more present with me during analysis than he had ever been.

One of the memories about him I described to Denae was a story told to me by my aunt, Dad's younger sister. Apparently, a fire had started in Dad's parents' three-story home, and Dad dashed up the smoke-filled stairway to rescue me, his two-year-old daughter, who was napping upstairs.

The fire was common knowledge in family history, but it wasn't until I was an adult that it became curious to me that we had never talked about how the fire started. Some fifty years after the event, I asked Dad if he knew what started the fire. Much to my surprise, he was willing to discuss the cause and actually seemed a bit relieved to be asked.

He admitted, in a straightforward manner that again surprised me, that he had hung his denim overalls on a poker near the fireplace. The poker had recently been used to stoke the fire.

He said he did not realize it was hot enough to catch his clothes on fire, a fire that spread enough to burn down part of his parents' home. Evidently, he felt so guilty about his mistake that he didn't speak of it for many years. He stuffed his feelings inside himself. At least that's my professional opinion about what happened based on knowledge gathered through my professional reading.

For him, it must have seemed safer to keep all his emotions buried, all but the festering anger that came out as irritation. Rather than modeling for me the normal human reactions of fear or anger, guilt or sadness, he showed me what shutting down looked like, stuffing one's emotions, displacing one's anger. It was all so clear to my psychologically trained conscious mind. What was hidden to me—and therefore keeping me stuck in the maturity level of a child—was that I was leading my own version of that life, putting out of reach all the wisdom the analyst was offering about contacting my feelings. Wisdom I might have integrated if it was not for my fear of sliding into a trench of overwhelming feelings, feelings I felt were dysfunctional.

As I was growing up, it was common for Dad to leave his field work, stomp into the house, sit down at the table, eat, and then go back outdoors to continue working. We did not ask him questions about what he was doing because he was usually gruff when he answered. We thought the gruffness was anger, and we had picked up that Mom was afraid of anger. So we stayed fearful of anger. And of him.

I was more able to approach him after Mom died (when I was an adult), and, somehow, my mind deleted the Dad of my childhood, the one I was afraid of, and replaced him with the dad I had wanted so I didn't have to feel the yearning of a child for her father. But through analysis, I began to realize how well he had taught me defenses against emotions, including the defense of repression of my childhood memories of him. At weak moments during my years of analysis, I wondered if my dad's way of dealing with emotions by hiding them might be easier than the path I was choosing. Maybe it *was* ridiculous spending so much money and time on analysis.

My dad was not the only person who showed me by example the value of repressing emotions. In the Midwest rural society in which I grew up, emotions were usually hidden. Feelings were believed to be, well, ridiculous.

I was well into analysis before I realized such self-control and walling-off of the emotional part of life was not necessarily a good thing. I think, now, about those three interconnected habits of mind—needing to feel I was a peer with adults, especially professionals in my field, being an avid reader so I could convince myself that I was smart enough, and justifying my behavior so I could remain where I was and not go through the pain of change.

These patterns managed to work independent of each other or in conjunction with one or both of the others. And how impossible it was for me for years to crack through that triumvirate of defenses so that I could go deeper.

─────

But what I really wanted Denae to tell me, was what it meant when I kept using Dad's word *ridiculous* again and again, which somehow morphed into wanting to know about the lights. Would she ever own up to buying new lamps? "This is ridiculous," I muttered.

Later I learned (through my readings) that the practice by an analysand of repeating words, when noticed by an analyst, could be useful to the analyst as one way to discover how the past continued to be in the analysand's present. This was a psychoanalytic assumption with which I would eventually resonate because of its clarity. But this day, I was more consumed with getting what I wanted. I wanted to know whether I was right that the lamps were new! It seemed vitally important to me. Almost a matter of life and death.

Suddenly I remembered a phrase I had run across, the almost alliterative phrase: the past is in the present; the past permeates the present. Remembering this bumper-sticker-worthy phrase, I uttered it aloud. I knew it had helped me develop respect for scraps and fragments of memory when they surfaced. They were the gold nuggets that would lead me to the rich veins of memory. In this reverie, the idea that appreciation of memory was the single greatest accomplishment of psychoanalysis (Chernin, 1995) also came to mind. I did not share the second gem because Denae seemed unimpressed with my first offering. The session came to a close with me feeling no clearer about my attraction to Dad's word *ridiculous* or whether the lamps were recent additions.

On my own, as I tried to understand more about myself and why sessions were so complicated and frustrating, I decided to look into my past to learn about the present situation. I felt I was applying my psychoanalytic knowledge when I dug out the journal entry I made after my first analytic session on October 1, 2007. I was surprised with what I found. Shocked, actually. I had written these phrases, which were uncharacteristically floating on the page: "found out something going on under the surface," "out of control," "intense, willing and able to dip under the surface," "not someplace I've been able to go 'cause need to keep surface calm."

This entry puzzled me. Did this mean that I knew about repressed emotion way back then? If I knew this after the first session, why has analysis lasted for so many years? I could not have articulated it at the time, but I was having my first flash of insight into the amazing capability of the mind to blot out, cover up, or repress what it doesn't want us to know. So, I knew, but I did not know. How strange.

If I had known (I said that a lot those days) that the relationship with the analyst would be like no other relationship, I might have changed my expectations for the relationship sooner. But, because I did not realize that, and because I knew nothing about Denae personally, I would project all my own ideas and feelings and mistaken notions on her. She acted as a mirror for me. Looking in that mirror was like observing myself on a bad hair day, but I did not want to look.

In case you are having difficulty understanding what I was going through, let me share another session. Actually, I only remember the part when I suddenly, out of nowhere, heard my voice say, "I forgot your check in the car." This admission darted out of my mouth without my realizing I had even been thinking about the check or about paying her. She had been, it seemed to me, hinting around that I was not as responsible as I thought I was. It soon occurred to me, with a sense of irritation, that I had just proved her point.

She did not hesitate to point out: "Failure to pay attention to yourself can be seen as a lack of responsibility."

What would a parallel sound to her usual "Hmm" be? I needed such a sound right then. She was right about not paying attention to myself (though I never thought of that as being irresponsible), but I could see her point. And she was not done: "You didn't want to pay me."

What was she trying to say to me? I hesitated, not being aware enough to admit that no, sometimes I didn't want to pay her. Sometimes I didn't even like her. Sometimes I wanted to quit. But at that time, I could not allow myself to know any of that, so I argued with her, telling her that what she was saying was ridiculous (oblivious to the fact that I was using my father's word). That of course I wanted to pay her. Paying her was the responsible thing to do.

The session over, I went home baffled. I understood part of what she was saying, but not all. That would take more time. Lounging on my bed at home, I focused on old defensive questions. Did I really need to continue with psychoanalysis? I knew I was anxious, but wasn't everyone? I had fears, but I managed them (mostly). Just how messed up was I? I could handle almost anything, but still, was I defective? My life was rich and full and the longer I was in treatment, the better it became; but was there a causal relationship?

One Monday after reading journal entries that differed one from the other about what had happened in a particular session, a question was fresh in my mind: how or why do my notes have differing memories of the same incident? This was a legitimate concern I felt so I decided to bring it up to Denae as a question, of course, in a free association sort of way. It might foster discussion of psychoanalysis between two peers, but I was blissfully unaware of that hope.

I wish I could hug the naive woman I was when I attended this cloudy, windy Monday afternoon session. I entered the consultation room, which was darker than usual, and stretched out on the couch. I straightened the blanket over my legs to help distract me from reproaching myself for having already decided on a free association, when I knew it would be better to trust myself and see what came up. I began, as if it had just occurred to me: "I wonder what you think is going on when a person has several different memories of the same incident?" Silence was the immediate answer to my question.

I settled into the silence, and began listening to the wind, which temporarily distracted me. How treacherous was it going to be walking to my car? I remembered that I'd had to park farther out than usual. Would I be blown away? Would I be able to get the car door open? I felt a chill in my upper body, so I pulled my soft and fluffy puffer coat over the blanket.

I wasn't exactly surprised when she finally spoke, "What ideas do you have about why someone would have various memories?" If someone had asked me to predict what she would say, I might have guessed she'd say something similar—after all, I'd been seeing her for a number of years.

"Well," I said, "I guess it sounds like the person who remembers things in several different ways wasn't really paying attention."

"Hmm." I always was fascinated (and mildly irritated) when she made this sound. Today it irked me.

"I can't think of any other reason." This was my attempt to seduce her into responding and this time it worked (though I did not like what she said).

"I think it indicates a lack of responsibility."

Now I felt annoyed. Was she suggesting that I was irresponsible? If I was anything, I was a responsible person. I knew this to be true without a shadow of a doubt. It was one characteristic that I prized about myself.

Denae's charge that I was irresponsible confronted one of my deepest-held beliefs about myself: I am a responsible adult. I am an oldest child. I had studied Murray Bowen's theory of birth order regarding personality, and I knew I followed the script that said oldest siblings were over-responsible and liked to be in charge, liked to call the shots. I know I have always been responsible.

It took months and much journaling for me to figure out that I had used study and knowledge to brand myself as mature and responsible. That was, in my mind, a non-negotiable truth. I justified my actions with the faulty reasoning of this truth. I knew I was a responsible person, and this firm belief prevented me from detecting problems in my behavior. This pattern of thinking I was blameless remained unconscious until it was brought to my consciousness by my analyst at a time when I had enough courage to see and accept that I did follow the pattern my analyst described—I was not always responsible.

Many times, my discovery of these unconscious patterns took place during very uncomfortable interactions with Denae. The chipping off of my certitude, like caked mud from a tire, was a long-drawn-out process. I clung to beliefs about my identity that had been in place for most of my life. When I began to learn about my unconscious patterns through analysis of my free associations, I began questioning the ways I had always thought about myself.

One of those unconscious beliefs, made possible by my third habit of mind—the ability to rationalize or justify anything—was this: if I asked for something from someone, that person should give it to me. I believed this was what I deserved because I did not ask for very much. I thought of myself as someone who took care of others. Of course, this was not a conscious belief. And I wasn't aware of the unconscious bargain I had made with the world: I will take care of you and I won't bother you by asking for what I need unless I really need it; in return, when I really need something, you should give it to me. This strategy, which I thought was just how good people behaved, had worked well for me. For the most part, I did not ask, and when I did ask, I received; so my justification for believing that people should give me what I wanted was reinforced.

A good example of how this belief worked in my mind can be demonstrated in the scenario surrounding one of Denae's planned absences. Denae was going on vacation (at least I assumed it was vacation because she told me the dates she would be out of the office). As she often did, she used my reaction (in this case, my reaction to her pending absence) as a psychoanalytic lesson. The following is what I remember.

"Here's a sheet listing the days I will be out of the office," offered Denae.

"Thanks, Denae. Where are you going?" I asked this as we walked across the room to take our places, me on the couch, she in a chair placed at the head of the couch so I could not see her. Silence. I started to feel sort of shy about asking when she was not forthcoming with an answer, so I began the session with another topic. In other words, I steered my associations away from the question and the session that unfolded was unremarkable. I left, clutching the paper in my hand, eager to mark these dates on my calendar.

We met for another session and neither of us raised the issue. But when we met for the following session, I began by sharing the following with her:

"I wrote in my journal that I was proud of being able to ask you forthrightly where you were going on vacation."

"How did that feel?"

"The session you informed me you were going to be out of the office, I was able to get to the place where I was trusting that you would tell me if you wanted me to know where you were going and that we would work it out. And that felt really good. But then I couldn't hang onto the trust I had in you and in our relationship and the trust that knew everything was going to be okay."

"And how did that feel?"

"Soon it was like I didn't even want to know where you were going! I didn't care! I was angry. I wanted to cut off from you! And all these feelings are so strange because I didn't really know why I was so upset."

It was difficult to tell her these feelings, especially the one where I wanted to cut off from her. She responded:

"You trusted me enough to tell me."

I felt a tear well up in my eye, but by the time I replied, I was dry-eyed. "It feels like I've had an emotional experience—like I've had a disaster or a loss. You are going to be gone for two weeks. I want to know where you are going on vacation. I feel there is only one right way for you to respond to my request."

"Hmm," she murmurs her neutral wordless response.

I continue, "Because of how you dealt with me, I have become aware of how I present things in an all-or-nothing way. I ask and unconsciously believe that, because I don't ask easily or often, I deserve the answer or whatever it is I request. I frame things in an all-or-nothing way so that if the other disagrees, she is wrong and in trouble with me. And I'm mad!"

She was silent as I continued talking, now, mostly to myself.

"This leaves no room for the other person to be separate and independent. It makes sense when I switch it around. If someone asks me something and I refuse to answer, it may mean I have a different reference point than that person, and, because of my separateness and independence, I need to refuse the request."

She held the silence for me to continue.

"I still feel a little mad at you, actually, but now it's not so much that I don't know and more that I didn't get my way! Do I actually deserve to know? Not really. I'd like to know but it's really okay that I don't."

After my longer-than-usual sharing, and another moment of silence, she said very quietly, "I feel protective of the space we have created together."

This felt new. Had I not been obsessing on needing an answer, I might have noticed that Denae had, at last, opened herself to me, referred to us as partners, creating something together. Exactly the kind of comment I had been yearning for, but I was so caught in my frustration, I heard it but didn't take it in. At least not then. The session drew to its usual close and I shuffled out the door.

That night, I noted in my journal that she thwarted me for several sessions and that I never found out, but this time it was not because I didn't ask. I kept repeating to myself that because of her stubborn refusal to not tell me where she was going, I learned about myself. I learned about my feelings of entitlement, and my way of researching things and then framing them as right or wrong so that the other person was either wrong or right by my standards. I learned that I didn't want to be that way, and I learned that the only way to not feel entitled was to recognize it when it happened.

It was halfway into the first week of her absence before I savored her parting words; I finally heard in the words she gave me that she was not going to tell me where she was going or anything else about her life, but that she was on my side. I repeated to myself her words, "I feel protective of the space we have created together."

Could it be that she kept her private life from me for my sake? She had seen how I wanted to merge with people, but also how I felt competitive with them and wanted to know all about them. She also had seen how I operated when I wanted something. It had taken me years to notice the subtle and clever ways I set about getting what I wanted. Would it take years more to undo that habitual behavior? Or would I find some way to rationalize it and justify it—a skill at which I excel.

8

STUBBORNLY STILL SPECIAL

At the risk of boring you, my reader, with more stories of my refusal to begin taking responsibility for my own behavior, I continue on, thinking it might be the only way for you to understand how deep and intractable was my need to think of myself as special, educated—not your ordinary analysand, but a bit above the rest.

"I noticed you had a big smile on your face when I greeted you. What was it like when I didn't return it?"

Initially, my bodily response to this unexpected question from Denae was to wrinkle my nose. It didn't seem like a real question. I hated it that she began our session that way. It was geared to make me admit that I felt hurt and it pissed me off. I thought to myself, there is no easy way to answer her. It sounded like a technique from Counseling 101 to me. Part of me wanted to snap back at her and tell her that I did not even notice she had not smiled. That might hurt her feelings and at that moment, I didn't care.

My good girl persona quickly appeared and cajoled me to take the high road, be nice, and hear the question in a positive light. This good girl (a label the analyst and I had begun using) was well instilled in me. So well instilled that, in fact, only recently had I come to understand that what I consider an accurate definition of myself—helpful, thoughtful, competent, reasoned, loving, inquisitive, kind—was not so much a description of me as it was the description of the persona I attempted to present to the world. That persona worked very well for me.

My inner adolescent (who also was trying to find a voice) and my good girl persona engaged in fierce struggles. My rebellious adolescent— the part of me that dug in my heels whenever Denae spoke, the little rebel who undercut any possibility I could respond to Denae maturely, so she could do what she was doing and that it would help me—that rebel smacked down the good girl and took charge.

"I will not speak! She cannot make me," my misguided teen declared, shouting into one ear.

At the same time, my good girl butted in and asked: "Did I smile when Denae stuck her head into the waiting room to greet me?" I honestly do not remember. And what does it mean if I did?

I remembered driving to her office debating which free association I was going to present and, as usual, not noticing the irony in my thought process. For me to use the technique of free association correctly, I would have had to say whatever came to mind in the moment. According to Freudian theory, this was a way to tap into the unconscious. Initially, I had imagined it would be easy to do, but it was far more difficult than I thought. Because I couldn't totally turn off my own profession, my inner therapist wanted to say things that Denae would find interesting and evocative. So, I chose and judged my ideas for free association ahead of time.

That all this made no sense and was a waste of time scarcely entered my mind. So, I fretted in advance, questioning all my ideas for free association until all that was left was the responsibility to say something. For years, Denae almost never got from me anything that could be called free association.

I have a flashback. One day early on in our work together, she disappointed me by refusing my request to start our sessions ten minutes past the hour (in other words, start the fifty-minutes of the psychoanalytic hour not on the hour but ten minutes after). I wanted to attend a Tai Chi class, and this would make it possible to do both the analytic session and the class without missing anything. Tai Chi seemed vital to my wellbeing because of my osteoporosis; the doctor's prediction was that, if I fell, I would break a bone. The analyst's cooperation seemed essential to my wellbeing, now and in the future. It was unfathomable to me when she refused my request.

I had read that people who used the confession booth learned by trial and error what to present to priests. They learned to reveal only those shortcomings that would not annoy the priests (which of course also meant the parishioners would not be made to feel uncomfortable by annoyed priests). I understood their strategies. I was doing the same thing during analysis to keep the analyst happy. But, like the parishioners who did not feel released from unconfessed sin, I was never able to be helped to change. And to compound my naivety, I convinced myself that Denae wasn't aware I was not freely associating.

When she did not return to her question about my smile, which I believe is an acceptable analytical move for her style of analysis, silence persisted. As the silence continued, I returned in my mind to her question of how it was for me when she did not return my smile. I began to wonder what I was smiling about, but I knew that what I was smiling about was not the point of her question. Her question, designed to encourage my expression of feelings, felt like pressure. Sure, I wanted to learn to express my feelings, but today?

I decided to change the subject. The rest of the hour was nondescript.

During another session, my immediate thought upon entering the consulting room was how much prettier Denae would be if she combed her hair. For years, I had had a fixation on her hair. Why wouldn't she want to look better while at work? I recalled the care I took to always look my best for my clients. I felt it showed respect for them.

I was learning to question my fixation on her hair, but it had been a struggle.

I shared with her how her ponytail reminded me of how Mom liked to pull my hair back into a ponytail. "My ponytail was my trademark when I was young," I boasted.

Thinking the interchange was going quite well, I kept it going. Inwardly it seemed as if perhaps at long last we were going to engage in *intersubjectivity*, psychotherapy jargon for relationships between people in contrast to individual experience. Early on, I proudly used this word to show my knowledge of psychoanalysis. She always went on as though she hadn't heard me. I was not going to say the word again, but perhaps we were doing it. I could only hope. It could mean that she was engaging with me more as a peer. My excitement led to mentioning how my hair was neatly pulled back.

Somehow contemplating the word neat led to voicing my opinion that her hair looked messy. I had noticed she was using a naked rubber band—like what is used to secure newspapers for delivery—on the top of her head to control some of her hair. Not a color-coordinated hair tie like my mother used for my ponytail. It looked ridiculous how her hair stuck straight up. I mean, come on—it was totally obvious that it was a mess. I was just telling the truth.

I was not at all prepared for her next remark.

"You like to be mean to me."

Oh my gosh—how was I going to get out of this? Had I really said that her hair looked ridiculous? I must have. I did not mean to, but it was the truth, and hadn't she encouraged me or at least implied that I was to be honest and say what came to my mind? Wasn't that free association? I rationalized my unkind judgmentalism.

The words "You like to be mean to me" were suspended in the stale psychoanalytic air. I realized uneasily that I was face-to-face with myself, as well as with the analyst. It became obvious I did have a part of me that could be mean, especially when I was feeling threatened. I had quickly assumed the stance of being above it all, untouched by normal human emotions. If there was a judge and jury present, I would have been convicted of both pride and arrogance before the hour was over. I had not admitted these character defects before that moment, because I had not recognized them as defects. I thought of them as honesty. This rationalization I had tried to keep hidden, especially from myself.

Suddenly, I realized I had the same type of subtle meanness that I had seen in my Dad and that I was so critical of. He was fond of calling other people ridiculous, based on their actions or emotions. And he did so in a way that seemed mean to me. So, when Denae said, "You like to be mean to me," I was shocked.

Quickly, I decided I did not want to think about my meanness and so changed the subject.

Expressing admiration seemed a way to appease her after being mean about her hair style. So I gushed about how much admiration I had for her because she did not waste time on her appearance. Those words sounded like a compliment until they were voiced. Maybe compliments were not appropriate in this case. I continued to think about her looks: she really must have cared about how she looked because she wore expensive-looking black knee-high boots. Anyone who wears boots is fashionable in my book. I felt like a stylish psychotherapist when I wore my boots at my office, though they were not as tall or as expensive-looking as Denae's.

"You don't like to think about your meanness."

She was not going to let this go. She knew she was right, that I had an underhanded way of being mean, often accompanied by laughter. She had worked with me long enough to recognize when my meanness arose. This was not the first time I had done something like that to her. She would continue to harp on my meanness until—I did not know when! What was I going to do? I did not think of it until later, but I could have just said that I recognized my mean part and apologized and asked her what I could do to make amends. But my ego was not flexible enough for me to think of that then.

Before analysis, I thought I was one of the nicest people you would ever meet. I thought I took care of others; I cared about others. I was a licensed social worker and licensed marital and family therapist, which to me, in effect, meant that I was trained to be nice. I went to church. I gave to the homeless. If the traffic would allow, I would pull over and give money to the scary-looking man holding a sign asking for help. But deep down, I knew she was right, I could be mean.

But it was hard to admit to myself that, unconsciously, I wanted to be mean to her. I strongly resisted having to think of myself as vindictive. There must be some other way of interpreting this behavior. It was more comfortable believing I was one hundred percent nice, and that it was only other people who acted mean. Just as I was beginning to hide behind my favorite rationalization—my honesty is helpful to others in the long run—the analyst said, "Our time is up for today."

As time went on, by staying faithful to professional rules, Denae helped me claim parts of myself that I didn't want to know. She taught me, without saying it out loud, that when I knew my deep feelings and desires, I had more control of when or how or if they came into view. But, for obvious reasons, I was uncomfortable moving into that unknown part, when, for almost six decades, I had felt safe being the nice girl persona I convinced myself I was.

During one session, Denae said something like, "You don't stay with your feelings long enough to get conviction about them. When you rush away from them, they don't have 'you' in them."

Was she correct? Probably. By quickly disregarding the shame and guilty conscience I might have had for hurting her and substituting pride for my being strong enough to be honest, I could feel good about myself without taking the time to really know what I had been feeling. To know my feelings, I would have to slow down and be present to the experience and acknowledge what I felt, even when that knowledge made me uncomfortable.

She was not finished.

"You seek approval to know it is okay to want something."

I remembered how Mom affirmed and appreciated every feeling I had. In some sense, Mom may have lived through me, taking my successes and accomplishments as her own. I felt anger toward her; anger and disappointment. If she had just… But then I stopped.

I remembered telling Denae that my experiences felt as if they did not really happen until I told Mom about them. But that was not Mom's problem; that was mine. I needed to be close to her. To, in a sense, feel her heartbeat. As I look back, I realize that recognizing this was my first step toward understanding how entwined I was with my mother, as if I was still connected to her by the umbilical cord.

Had I put Denae in the role of mother, which would mean, according to Freudian lore, that I was trapped in repeating the past in ways that kept me stuck in the present?

I purposefully did not share details with anyone regarding my secret life of psychoanalytic treatment. I mostly remained mute—fearful that others would ask the reasons behind this enormous outlay of time and money—and I was not sure how to explain my rationale.

It was hard to know what Danae thought was wrong with me, what my "issues" were. But, when I had an inkling that she thought I always wanted to be comfortable, frankly I had trouble seeing how this was a problem. In addition, I understood she believed that I did not feel my feelings, but I did not agree with her there either. Of course I felt feelings, I fumed to myself. I could not understand why she kept contradicting and challenging every picky little thing I said.

Why would she keep trying to make me mad, I wondered? I could not bear to describe these interactions to anyone. She made me feel defective, though, as a therapist, I knew that no one can make you feel anything.

We have a choice how to feel, I knew. But she made me so mad sometimes, I fumed, again not seeing the irony in my statement. The thought of telling someone anything about the whole endeavor brought down a shroud of shame that enveloped me. I felt sure everyone else knew what she was nudging me to accept. People might question my sanity if I told them how she spoke to me. I would learn later that there was a universal component to the flaws she was pointing out in me, but my omnipotent self-absorbed inner toddler was not able to comprehend this, let alone integrate her guidance.

The first few times I arrived for sessions, I was surprised she did not have the office prepared for me. For a few weeks, foremost on my mind was the issue of the waiting room radio being turned up so loud that it distracted me when we were in session. "I'm having trouble concentrating with the music so loud."

"You feel distracted."

"Yes, that's right. I can't concentrate."

"It is difficult for you to concentrate."

"Yes – is there anything we can do about it?"

"Do you have any ideas?"

"I think if you turned it down so it wasn't so loud, I would feel better."

"You think that my job is to make you comfortable?"

I seethed. This led to a discussion of how my need for comfort was interfering with my ability to enjoy life. I thought that making yourself and your loved ones comfortable was the thing to do, but she did not agree.

I honestly cannot explain how intense my level of frustration became during interchanges like these. Not many relationships in my history came close to duplicating the intense irritation I felt towards this analyst. And when I attempted to express my frustration, she would say:

"You seem irritated at everyone."

And some days she was correct. Some days, I did not like anyone. On those days, I knew that no one understood me. Whatever I said to her was turned back on me. She was not at all concerned about my comfort level. I could not believe it. She said things like, "You seem to have a lot of trouble with the blanket," or "No, I don't have any water available."

My relationship with Denae continued to be intense while, surprisingly, the rest of my life became more relaxed and comfortable. Was there a correlation?

Occasionally during my first two years of treatment, the door to the whole building where

Denae had her office would be locked when I arrived for my session. One time, my cell phone was in the car so I returned to the parking lot and called her so she could unlock the door. An indistinguishable mix of strong feelings welled up inside me when I put my hand on the door handle and it did not budge.

I mostly was able to forgive her when she told me that other tenants in the building were responsible for locking the door. Whether I was eagerly awaiting my appointment that day or dreading it, I found the shock of being shut out was traumatic. My mind said I was overreacting, but my feelings were hurt. And, of course, it felt too petty to reveal these feelings.

During one of the sessions, when I had been locked out of the building, I reported to her for no particular reason that I asked my osteopath if I could rest on the table for a few minutes to let the treatment integrate into my body.

Denae's response was unexpected: "You like feeling special."

These words, with the further implication that I was accustomed to feeling special, were words that hurt the most of all the observations Denae had made. I did like feeling special and I found it hard to understand why she thought there was a problem with wanting to feel special.

Later in the session she said, "You liked staying at the doctor's as long as you wanted."

I could not swear to what she was trying to accomplish by saying that, but I inferred it was something about me needing to be special. When I questioned her, why? she replied in a very even tone, "You didn't want me to say that." Frustration mounted.

I took a deep breath and sighed, taking the stance of the adult with an unreasonable child: "Let me explain." And I went on to slowly clarify my intention. "I wasn't trying to feel special; I was trying to be adult, taking responsibility for my own needs by asking the doctor for extra time. I had had to learn how to be assertive years ago during the women's movement." And then, not wanting her upset with me, I rationalized. She couldn't have known this. She was young and grew up reaping the rewards of the Women's Movement I had had to fight for. I could forgive her ignorance.

I had become so good at rationalization that it didn't matter that there were logical holes in my thinking. All I had to do was apply a general diagnosis onto every problem without ever thinking through whether it applied or not and I would feel better.

Much later, I realized that, when it came down to it, I was hard pressed to find anything she did that I could claim was sexist. I had no way of knowing that her observations were designed, as part of the analytical process, to irritate me and send me deeper and deeper into examining my own motivations. In time they would serve as vehicles for my transformation.

Over many sessions, it had started to become clearer to me that Denae wanted me to understand that being the center of attention, feeling entitled (being above it all), and feeling special put me at risk of never growing up completely. She wanted me to realize that, when I faced something scary and I responded by thinking that the scary or bad thing should not be happening to me, it was impossible for my unconscious to use that event to help me grow up. When I focused on the unfairness of the scary or bad thing, I did not create any fixes. Instead, I just gave up.

I was lying on the couch, contemplating how true all those patterns of mine were, but not liking to admit any of them. I knew the session was almost over (I have a sixth sense about how long fifty minutes is). I always made her say that the time was up. I figured it was her job to set the closing boundary. There was no clock on the ceiling, and if I peeled off the blanket and pushed up my sleeve to look at my watch, she would see me do it. I did not want her to know that I was wondering how much time was left. I could count on her to wait until the very last minute and then say curtly, "Our time is up for today." I got up and left, knowing how unresolved the session had been, and how glad I was to have it over.

When I got to the car and opened my notebook, I started taking notes on what had happened. A scene popped into my mind of one day when I was in my thirties, and Mom asked if she and Dad could bring some of their friends over to my house on Sunday afternoon. I was caught off guard and immediately thought of how that was the time my husband and I set aside to be together, so I said, simply, "No."

Her visceral response was, "How dare you?" And she began listing all the things she had done for me since I was born. Now, my angry feelings toward Denae spread to my mother, and, oh how I hated them both.

It took a few days for me to realize what was likely abundantly clear to Denae—I was not the easiest client for her to deal with. How could she get past my need to be her peer or even friend, my questioning of her methods, and my penchant for planning my spontaneity. How could she help me realize that I was not working toward my own health, which was the whole point of analysis?

And then I couldn't help but feel a little special in my obstinacy.

9

SHE LOVES ME MOST

Nina, the sister who disrupted my only-child life when I was six, and my other less disruptive sister Nan, who appeared on the scene when I turned ten, cleaned out the attic of my father's home after he died, in preparation for a garage sale. Between the two of them, they saved almost everything, and boxed it up to cart to their homes, so my involvement in the mice-infested attic was zero. Nina continued to sort through boxes of memorabilia for months, and because Nina knew what to save for me, I had all the treasures I wanted without putting in any effort on the project.

I did not often speak of my siblings when I lay on the analytical couch because, truthfully, I did not think of them that often and almost never in terms of how to understand my mind, which was the purpose of psychoanalysis. I was always surprised when Denae remembered details about them. She heard the most about Nina, and not as much about my brother Nolan, who was born a year after Nina. She seemed to know about my sister Nan, who, as I mentioned, was born ten years after I was, and Nyla, the youngest, who was born fifteen years after my birth.

Because I had told Denae about the attic cleaning effort, I could not wait to share the details of the contents of the envelope Nina had found in the attic and mailed to me. It contained letters I wrote to my mother when she was in the hospital giving birth to Nina. I did not know of their existence and had no memory of having written them. It was discombobulating to see my innocent-looking six-and-a-half-year-old printing. I used the salutation: "Dear Mama." How odd. I don't ever remember calling Mom *Mama*. The first line of the note was a short but telling sentence: "I'm fine."

It seemed odd to me that, when I was separated from Mom, my main caretaker, my first thought when writing her was one of reassurance. I was okay. These unasked-for and unsought-after pieces of paper from the past provided evidence for what my analyst had previously speculated: at one time in my life, I felt adored and adored my mother and felt I had to take care of her.

The charming childish handwriting continued: "I've been playing 'Doctor Doctor' on the piano." This bit of detail was a clue that I was staying with my paternal grandparents while my mother was in the hospital. Grandma Carrie's piano was her prized possession; she was a trained piano instructor.

I saw this note as evidence regarding the quality of the relationship Mom and I enjoyed before she gave birth to more children. I also thought this short and sweet note made our relationship sound like we were lovers, not mother and daughter, because I needed to reassure her. She was away. I was okay. I would wait for her. My implied but unstated assumption was that we would go back to the way things were when she returned—which of course was a big mistaken notion on my part.

During the next analytical session, after I talked about the notes I had written to my mom, I decided to tell the analyst a dream from the night before, in which I was backing down the driveway very fast while singing, "Dora Dora." When I finished describing the dream, I said that I had no idea what it meant. But in this particular session, unlike what usually happened during my sessions, I kept thinking of the dream and did not cut myself off. The couch felt safer than usual, so I allowed an honest-to-goodness free association: "I have not one, but three baby books. Books that Mom filled out only partially." The associations kept coming: "I wrote a blog post on the idea that what is behind you is as important as what is in front of you. I wrote this without being conscious of the fact that this is what I am doing in psychoanalysis!"

This is working, I mused to myself. I am going to access my feelings. But then, my impatience regarding how everything was taking so long surfaced and I began to feel despondent. I said, without thinking about it (another true free association), "I want to get out of there. I do not want to do analysis anymore!"

"You want to block this out," observed Denae.

"Yes, it's my three-year-old self. No, it's my two-year-old self."

"Why two?"

"Because I acted like a two-year-old just now!"

Long pause. I asked a question, despite knowing the chances were slim I would receive an answer: "Do you think I was acting like a two-year-old?

"I don't think the best way to get to know a feeling is by what age it is," she replied.

Okay.

I discerned she was right and that I needed to try and stir up and capture and express the elusive feelings I ordinarily repress, feelings I was beginning to think just might be present. I was impatient. It felt like I was being picked on. I really did not want to do analysis anymore. Desperate to not feel that out of control, I started to think of what I would have for lunch. Interrupting my menu planning she inquired: "What did you write to your mother when Nina was born?"

"Oh!" I responded with a shudder of recognition. "I said, I am fine. I'm fine. So I have been saying that I was fine since I was six years old. I was fine. I would take care of everyone and everything. I wouldn't have feelings. I was fine."

I took a deep breath. "I feel so sad."

Denae said, "Maybe 'Dora Dora' was like 'Doctor Doctor,' the song you told your mother you played on the piano."

A feeling swept over me, an almost mystical sense, as if truth was in the air, surrounding me, permeating me, frightening me. "That could be right," I murmured.

Then, quickly I turned my focus to her and mentioned how impressed I was by how well she made such a great association. Or was that an interpretation? Whatever it was, I was not sure how knowing that 'Dora Dora' from my dream was related to 'Doctor Doctor' was helpful, except that it occurred to me it could be an indication that my unconscious was active.

Suddenly, I was curious about what I might have said in the note to my mom if I had told her the truth, though I couldn't say for sure what that truth would have been. And I also wondered what I would say if I stopped assuring the people now in my life that I was fine. Maybe that question is coming from my unconscious, my conscious mind speculated.

Denae had been insinuating for quite some time that I suppressed my anger. Or was it repressed? In other words, was I conscious of my anger enough to consciously press it out of consciousness because I didn't want to feel it? Or did I repress the anger before it ever had a chance to make it to my conscious mind? I clearly did not understand my anger. She had been trying to goad me into anger for a long time. She would say she wanted me to know and express the emotion of rage. Sometimes she pointed out that I was angry with her. I always vehemently denied her accusations, not wanting to give her the satisfaction of knowing she could make me angry.

Once, I had reasoned with her, "How could I be angry with you for being late to our session? After all, you were only a few minutes late. I know that sometimes things happen."

That didn't satisfy her. She continued, "But you looked upset when I met you in the waiting room. You are upset."

"Denae, you are usually on time and I appreciate that so much. I know I would hate to have to wait a long time. But I am not an unreasonable person. I'm a therapist too, and I know that things can happen."

Perhaps I was a little upset. But I didn't feel I was angry. She acted like it was an easy thing to get mad. She seemed to think it was very clear that there was something repressed that I needed to face. How could she be so sure when I was equally sure there wasn't?

⁓

The hardest part of analysis for me was to express emotions in front of Denae, especially anger. And I suspect that for Denae her challenge was to help me find, feel, and express anger. One day, I decided to tackle this in an analytical session with Denae but, as usual, I started out not saying what I really wanted to say. Instead I said, "I am really curious what is going to come up and out today."

There was silence.

"I have been feeling a really sad feeling but one I know I can handle." When I said this, I was thinking of my youngest son's recent comment that I then shared with her. He had remarked, "Mom, you had sad eyes in that picture by the Christmas tree."

More silence.

"I told him I didn't see my sadness. It pained me for him to say I was sad. I felt like he was criticizing me. I thought I was happy during that Christmas season while I was single."

"I don't disagree with you, but I think you are going quickly to fixing," Denae replied.

When she said this, I felt my belly becoming heavy and sluggish. It felt dark. I wondered what that meant? I wanted to tell her, so I said simply, "My belly feels empty."

"Can you say more?"

More silence.

"Now my belly feels full and busy. A lot is going on. I don't know what's happening!"

"You could get to know what's happening by waiting."

Thinking of my belly, I free associated to how embarrassed and horrified I was when I took Jon, a man I was dating, to a party with my friends and he wore a tee shirt that made his belly look huge. His belly protruded so much the shirt was too short to cover it. I whispered my dismay to one of my friends. She grinned at me and giggled, "I thought he looked cute!" I certainly did not agree but felt a tiny bit less critical while I remember wondering if she would say the same thing if it was her boyfriend.

Feeling that I really had a genuine free association, I decided to share this incident about bellies from the past with Denae. Soon, I regretted bringing it up. She kept hounding me with questions: What was it exactly about big bellies that I did not like? I could not believe we had to spend this much time on this example, since it had happened years ago.

Continuing her interrogation, Denae asked me if I remembered when Mom's body shape changed and what sort of reaction I had?

Imagining myself as a girl observing my mother's changing body shape was not easy but it was preferable to searching for words to describe the belly feelings I had shared with Denae that led to her current interrogation. Uncharacteristically, I opted to use my imagination and pictured the first time or two that Mom's belly grew large. It likely would have meant things were changing, which would have been a little frightening. I was happy with things the way they were. However, if I could be sure that Mom really wanted to be pregnant after Nina was born (Nina's birth was so easy in contrast to mine),

I would be able to picture Mom's brown eyes twinkling as she patted her belly and I looked on adoringly as she would have wanted. But, were there feelings I pushed down into my unconscious? Feelings that would have upset Mom?

The analyst interrupted my reverie to suggest that Mom's growing belly might have registered in my psyche as an indication of another rival on the horizon. I heard the implied message: In my mind, fat bellies were a threat. Having rivals took away from my special position. Lying there in Denae's office sixty-plus years later, I returned to thinking about my belly. It was still difficult to describe the feelings I was having. Surely, I thought, I'm not still worried about losing a singular place in my mother's heart.

10

MY BODY COMPLICATES EVERYTHING

One day, for no reason that I was conscious of, I found myself using the word *venture* to describe how I had been venturing into Freudian psychoanalytic treatment. Since the word *venture* came to me in a free-association (it was easier to free-associate off the couch sometimes), I felt compelled to look it up and discovered how appropriate the word was: a *venture* is an activity or undertaking involving risk or uncertainty because one cannot possibly see the destination.

No wonder my unconscious chose this word, I thought. While embarking on this adventure, I had never considered that Denae could—and, indeed would—move her office and do so without consulting me. I know, to many of you readers, this sounds hopelessly naïve—as if I assumed she saw my need for her to remain in the same office, as if I expected the whole world to be as I needed it to be.

I had taken the fact that her location—on the street where my psychotherapy internship supervisor had resided—was a psychoanalytic placard, a sign of connection for me that translated to an easy feeling in my body and soul. Minuscule travel time from home to this location added to my comfort. I admit that I did not recall this historical information every time I headed out for an appointment with her. After the first year, this connection scarcely entered my conscious mind. The unconscious ease, however, remained consistent until the upsetting news that she was moving.

An angst-filled journal entry in January of 2011, three years into my psychoanalysis with Denae, serves as my narcissistic commentary on this perilous (to me) relocation: "Go today to Denae's new office. I remember at our last session crying out in a childlike voice, 'I don't want you to move.' I haven't been writing as I feel too embarrassed to express what is on my mind and too frantic to slow down and figure out what is in my heart."

I don't doubt my journal entry, but I will confess with mixed feelings that I have no memory of the childlike crying out that I captured on the page. No doubt the analyst was pleased with my expression of emotion, though my lack of memory would not have pleased her. And it puzzled me. If expressing feelings was so vital to my wellbeing, it seemed to me that this crying out would have found a place in my memory.

"But you wrote it down," I heard a voice whisper from somewhere.

The building she was abandoning, one block from a heavily trafficked main road, offered parking directly in front. One day I had arrived early and witnessed Denae's late arrival. This meant that I had discovered something personal about her besides her naming story—the type of car she drove!

Her new office's building, surrounded by a parking lot edged with flowering trees, was off the main city streets. When I arrived for my first appointment at the new location, I looked for her car (as I always had since I found out what it was). I didn't see it, so, needing reassurance I had found the right location, I drove around the building.

There it was. I knew I had found her. As this new location was approximately five minutes farther from my home, I learned in time that the extra miles in the car usually provided more time for developing my free associations.

I know. That makes no sense. But it is an indication of how defended I was against her getting through to me on any deep level, how much in control I thought I needed to be. The whole idea and practice of free association violated my internal rules about what was safe, appropriate, and coherent to share with another person including my analyst.

While Denae did not (in my opinion) completely adhere to the stereotype of the Freudian analyst as an arid, stiff person who maintained an utterly impersonal atmosphere in the analytic session, she did not ask very many direct questions. This cultivated a feeling of formality. It felt to me as if she did everything she could to avoid influencing me, which sometimes I appreciated and other times I didn't. She remained courteous, and cordial, was at times gentle, and on rare occasions provided sincere empathic input. I understood why she consistently maintained the analytic attitude, but at times I thought it would have been helpful to know her perspectives. I was, after all, trying to emulate some of her techniques in my own professional work.

The first time I drove to the new office, I was anxious about finding the building, and ended up having very little planning time for free associations. I arrived unprepared and, obviously, was still largely unaware of the irony of planning my free associations ahead of time. Stepping into Denae's suite, I recognized most of the furniture from the old office. I perceived with pleasure that the radio was farther away from the consultation room. The distracting music would no longer interfere with my concentration.

But there were new issues. The consultation room featured a glaringly bright ceiling light which was directly in my line of sight when I took my supine position on the couch. I was incensed. How could she expect me to put up with that?

"That is the most irritating light I have ever seen!" I said, proud of myself for being upfront, but ashamed of my contentious tone.

"You don't like the light."

As I worked through this new aversion, I feared I was exhibiting some of the same qualities that popped out when I was trying to solve the interfering radio din in the former office. I was thankful that she did not resort to the blaming comment she used when I raised the issue of the loud music:

"It seems you are saying that I'm not providing the correct environment for you."

It turned out that the solution to the problem of the blinding light was fairly straightforward: turn it off when I passed by the switch on the way to the couch. When I took charge and turned off the light, I felt bossy and demanding.

A child with an inflated sense of self. Oh dear, was I being the person she had implied I was earlier? A strutting four-year-old? She would never comment on whether it was acceptable behavior on my part to turn off the light, but I decided that I would turn it off as I couldn't bear looking at the light.

Immediately, an annoying metaphor surfaced in my mind: "Nicky couldn't bear seeing the light concerning her own shortcomings." I decided this formulation was a ridiculous simplification, so I dismissed it. After all, I did not want to be one of those annoying people who make meaning out of everything.

My lessons in free association continued and appeared in various contexts. Before psychoanalysis I was not aware that random minuscule memories, stockpiled carefully in the brain, could be a pathway to the unconscious. I wished someone would have clued me in; it took me a long time to find out for myself that there are reasons we choose words or phrases to remember. Most of the time, the reasons are unknown because they are buried deep in the unconscious. It takes work to uncover their meaning. This, I was to learn, was a pivotal part of psychoanalysis.

I remembered a phrase I gleaned from a lecture for docents at the local art center: absence is presence. Initially, the surprising and somewhat paradoxical idea that absence can be presence made little sense to me. As a self-described commonsense person, I immediately tried to dismiss the idea. It made no sense especially when gazing at a work of art, but for some reason I wrote the phrase in big letters in my journal.

Much later, I began puzzling the merit of absence is presence, with its clouded meaning—a phrase I had stored in my unconscious for years following the docent lecture, a phrase I assumed must be brilliant. Absence is presence. At long last my consciousness penetrated an understanding of this phrase: Paying attention to what is no longer present or is unseen—to what a person thinks should be there but isn't—has value. I metaphorically saw the light! The phrase drifted deeper into my consciousness and morphed into a new phrase: absence of health is sickness. This seemed profound.

But why? Why was I proud of a thought that, on reflection, was obvious, not profound? And then it hit me. What was important was that I had mentally shifted from circuitous mental thoughts to noticing something about my body. It wasn't doing well. Strange symptoms were occurring. Not only was my body trying to get my attention, but even random activities of the day were drawing my attention to my body.

One day, while restless and rummaging through a musty box I had rescued from the lower-level storeroom of my home, I discovered seven of my grade school report cards, handwritten in ink on yellowing paper. I noticed the multiple absences, something I had often heard my parents mention: "You missed so much school, you almost weren't promoted to second grade."

Their observation was not an exaggeration. According to my report card, during kindergarten, I missed one third of the days and in first grade, I missed two thirds of the days. During these two years, my mother gave birth to my sister and my only brother. Close examination of the data—plus prompting by my analyst's question, "How did your mother feel when she got pregnant?"—fostered ideas that I hoped would encourage forward movement in my psychoanalysis, so I wouldn't have to be in analysis forever.

Questions such as: Did my illnesses have anything to do with Mom's morning sickness, or her giving birth to two children within fifteen months?

At the very least, it must have been a confusing time for me as a child of six. Two new babies, diapers to wash, bottles to sterilize, all tasks that can be overwhelming to a young mother. Mom had been my favorite playmate. Perhaps my illness was psychosomatic in nature? When mom needed me, I could be there, if ill enough to stay home. Or perhaps the illnesses garnered me her attention, which otherwise was focused elsewhere. As I waded further into the psychoanalytic arena, this type of layered thinking and speculation both puzzled and frustrated me. I liked things to be simple.

The most obvious but simplistic answer to the reason for my childhood illnesses was that I became ill so I could stay home with my mother and become her helper with the babies. Or perhaps I needed some care-giving energy from my mother that I was used to, attention that was now being showered on the babies. Or maybe I felt the need to control the interlopers as best as I could which would be the beginning of my life-long desire to be in charge.

When I was ill as a child, the green couch in our living room was where I spent time lying under a sheet tent-like structure with a steam vaporizer. My only chore was to rub Vick's under my nose. I didn't have to set the table. The couch was my safe haven as a child. As an adult, occupying the couch in the analyst's office was a different experience. While I was beginning to feel more psychologically comfortable on the couch after being in treatment for several years, my body began perplexing me. Strange symptoms appeared in my body and would not go away.

That was how I thought of it—"my body," like I would say, "my clothes," or "my purse." It was not really me. My left side hosted all the uncomfortable symptoms. My left foot would hurt if I did not wear very supportive, non-fashionable shoes. If I walked very far, my left hip would hurt and then the pain would run down my leg. I was no longer afraid of missing school, as I imagined I might have been when I was young, but now I was worried about missing work. I loved my work as a psychotherapist, and I cared a great deal about the welfare of my clients. I decided not to take new referrals for the foreseeable future and felt grateful my analysis still would fit in the budget. But to focus enough to capture and then express the thoughts needed for free association was exhausting. So many thoughts were present, I could not keep track of them. Which ones would I choose to express?

Sometimes when I spoke unguardedly to the analyst, I experienced the bodily sensation of dizziness on the top of my head, the physical part of my body closest to the analyst. I tried to console myself when the dizziness came by saying to myself that the only thing happening was thinking about an issue in a new way. I wanted to know the origin of the symptoms. Often, I neglected to mention these odd occurrences to her because they were difficult to explain. How could my thoughts make me dizzy? Was I going backwards in my analysis?

Even though I had questions, I did not want to express concern about my body in session. I had my own idea about what was causing most of my symptoms, especially when they first began. In addition to the dizziness described above, I had symptoms mostly related to my difficulty walking. The somatic therapist I had consulted for two years, at the suggestion of a massage therapist I trusted, focused on my posture, and as a result I truly was standing straighter. At least that was changing! It made sense to me that changing my center of balance and moving in a different way would take time to become natural, and that meanwhile I might be occasionally dizzy.

Several months later I experienced a much more serious health event while sitting in the car, as I attempted to pull my coat's belt from underneath my butt. As I tugged and twisted, an excruciating pain shot through my entire right side. The pain was so sharp and intense I could hardly breathe. Never had I felt a sensation so painful. For a few minutes, I wondered if I would be able to drive home. Luckily, the pain eased enough for me to place the car in reverse and back out of the space in the office parking lot. My husband's own back issues at the time would have prevented him from coming to collect me. I thought he had enough on his plate, so I didn't add to his worries by complaining about myself after I got home. The pain mostly went away the next day, so I did not worry about it.

I cringed thinking of confiding in my analyst and sharing my body aches. I must have believed with all my misguided brain power that I would not receive the type of empathy I wanted, so I barely mentioned the painful car incident to Denae. It was difficult for me to be vulnerable, though I did not know that consciously.

My symptoms, including a sense of agitation and anxiety, had not calmed down. My relationship with being sick, if that is what you would call what I was experiencing then, was very complicated. Because I was sick a lot as a kid, my analyst and I had talked about the possibility that this might have been a bid for attention when my mother started having other children, which might have seemed to me at the time like my mother breaking up with me.

I thought again of my absences from school and then wondered, where was I present during those years? I have almost no memories of either school or home. Surely, I should be able to remember when my sister or brother were brought home from the hospital or instances of them crying or Dad walking the floor with one or the other. My life had been disrupted, but I had no memory of any of my siblings coming home to expand the family. The only proof I had of my discomfort (because I did not remember any of the stories locked away in my unconscious) was a black and white deckle-edged photo of me wearing a mildly disgusted look while staring at an infant on wrinkled bed sheets.

Bessel Van Dan Der Kolk, M.D., in *The Body Keeps the Score* (van der Kolk, 2014), proposed that lack of memory may be related to trauma. Traumatized people simultaneously remember too little or remember too much, he wrote. There could be no undoing of the trauma, but what could be dealt with were the imprints of the trauma on body, mind, and soul. The example of such an imprint was feeling crushing sensations in the chest, which reminded me both of recent feelings on the analytical couch and of my childhood respiratory illnesses. My new symptoms did not include coughing repeatedly to purge phlegm as I had as a child, but I was not able to walk normally. And I was scared.

I couldn't count on my body anymore. I began feeling exhausted most of the time. I did not have my sense of balance; it felt as if I might fall over when I was in a crowd of people. I had to urinate frequently and was worried about the embarrassment of not making it in time to the restroom. I needed some answers about what was happening. One thing I knew how to do was to research through psychoanalytic books. Surely there would be an answer for me if I dug deep enough.

A sentence in a book on psychotic anxieties, almost made me cry, I felt so understood. In an introduction to her book, *Psychotic Anxieties and Containment*, Grotstein thanked Margaret Little, the author, for sharing her first-hand experience with what he termed:

> "...emotional depths many of us have either never had to traverse or never had sufficient guidance to be able to be conducted through such an inner Purgatory that we only dimly realized lay within us."
>
> (Margaret Little, 1990)

What touched me was Grotstein's acknowledgement of how the emotional depths faced in psychoanalytic treatment felt like Purgatory. When I heard the word Purgatory, angst and relief flooded my body. Grotstein went on to note that Little's account of her analytic experience was of special value since Little, too, was an analyst.

I was thrilled. Little was a therapist like I me! (Well, not exactly, but she worked with clients!) I dove into the text. The first sentence I underlined concerned an illness she and I had in common: pneumonia. Little said that pneumonia was part of an early breakdown she had at age five, and that it was brought about by massive sudden changes. I had pneumonia at around age five, during the time when I was experiencing massive changes: first, I had become aware of my mother's morning sickness and then my siblings began arriving. Suddenly I remembered something Denae had offered me: "You suffered a huge loss when you were five and six, didn't you?" I had dismissed it at the time probably because I thought the story was too ordinary. But now as I remembered it and felt unfathomable feelings, I think she might be right. I kept reading.

Little described a session with her analyst during, in which she experienced an infantile state. It was as if she heard my question, "What does that mean?" and answered with a description: bodily tension rising to a climax followed by relief, which were the same symptoms she described the fetus experienced before birth. As I was reading, I recalled experiencing feelings of tension in my belly, as well as feelings of dizziness, while on the analyst's couch. I was so interested in the relationship between my mind and my body, especially now that I was having all these bodily symptoms. Could analysis be causing my symptoms? Could it cure them?

What can I do to figure out what is causing all these symptoms?

Because books were my go-to for comfort and information, and because I believed they could help me, I asked my analyst to recommend a book on psychoanalysis—a reasonable request, I thought, especially in light of the short stack of books I saw on a desk in the consultation room. I fantasized she would pick up a big thick one and handing it to me say, "Take this home and we will discuss it next week." Instead, the conversation unfolded like this:

"Would you please recommend a book on psychoanalysis to me?"

"Why are you asking me for a book?"

"I want to know more about psychoanalysis, especially psychosomatics."

"What will you do with the information?"

Oh my. This was complicated, like everything I brought up with her. I just wanted her to give me a book recommendation! What was so hard about that?

She asked, "Do you think that reading about psychoanalysis will help you?"

"Yes, I do think it will help me. Books have always helped me."

"You would rather read than be here experiencing psychoanalysis."

I mumbled (mostly to myself) that I could do both. Clearly, she was not going to recommend a book. Confused and disappointed, I silently decided to continue finding my own damn books. Since I loved following the threads that led from one book to another and yet another, that was not a huge problem. But why would she not answer my question with an answer, not another question? That was all I was asking for. An answer!

11

All I Ever Wanted Was the Oceanic Feeling

When I was going through my divorce and then newly single, I did not have the words *oceanic feeling* to describe what I believed had been missing and what I longed for. I only knew I wanted a relationship with a man who shared my spirituality, who needed me even as I needed him, and with whom I could merge, a merging that would involve sexuality, but would be more than that. Deeper than that. It would involve being swept away by another, diving into another's world, drowning in another's attention and love, floating on another's strength—all a part of what I now know can be described as an oceanic feeling. This deep, unarticulated desire in one form or another had guided my actions for much of my life, affecting my spirituality, driving my sexuality, and adding a layer of difficulty to all my close relationships. I needed too much and had unrealistic ideas of what was possible.

When reflecting on how this need affected my spirituality, I realized before analysis there was never a question in my mind as to whether God existed. I knew He did, based on feelings of oneness I had sometimes experienced, feelings that were almost orgasmic in their intensity, as if my whole body yearned to be enveloped, like the pure sensory experience of floating in warm, sustaining water.

A memory surfaced. I was ten years old, kneeling at the chancel rail of my picturesque rural United Methodist church, remembering what had happened the night before in a half-dream and half-awake state: the tingles, the build-up, the rush, the enveloped feeling. I had wanted the feeling never to end until I remembered cuddling with my mother as a small child and seeing the disappointed look on her face when I began to touch myself. I do not think she said anything as she disentangled us, but she put me down quickly and left the room. Uncertain what the problem was, I believed I had done something wrong.

While kneeling at the rail in church, I prepared for communion by asking God to forgive me—for what, I wasn't sure, and then I prayed for the special feeling I craved, because if God gave it to me, it couldn't be wrong. I determined it was most likely that God would give me that rush while I was in this kneeling posture. I believed the closer my body was to the front of the church, where the holiness took place, the more likely God would grant my wish.

On this communion Sunday, I exposed my left palm so the minister could place on it the flattened piece of what I secretly called Wonder bread right in its middle to rest until we were instructed to eat. The minister made another pass down the rail, this time holding a shiny metal round container with a layer of thimble-sized glasses of grape juice. Responsible eldest that I was, I wondered who would have to wash all these tiny glasses. As I waited for the rush of feeling, I surreptitiously peeked up at the colorful round stained-glass window of Jesus kneeling in the garden. He and I were sharing the same humble posture. That must mean something. I began to feel holy, important, and special. I waited. And waited, remaining on my knees, while I heard the sounds made by other worshippers as they stood in order to return to their pews. I felt brave and bold. But, the more I focussed on that part of my body, the secret place where the rush begins, the more I realized it was not going happen. Maybe I had done something wrong.

I returned home, disappointed but hopeful that maybe, when communion was served again, that feeling I loved would come with the grape juice and bread. I stretched out in my father's musty smelling canvas hammock, a relic from his time in the Navy. Staring up through the leaves, into the clouds, breathing the fresh air, I began to feel unique, connected to nature, and safe. I moved my body to produce a rhythmic swing to the hammock. Then, I touched myself tenderly, needing to believe that all these feelings were evidence of God's presence. Of God's love. Of God's desire that I would be embraced, that I would be immersed in this powerful sensation, that it would bring me certainty that I was singularly loved.

Then I sensed the presence of Mother, her eyes filled with fear, or maybe it was disappointment. The feeling of being enveloped in love vanished as I popped open my eyes. No one was there. Quickly, I closed my eyes again, swaying with the hammock, praying for that feeling to return, the feeling of being enveloped and safe. Nothing. I waited. Still nothing. Never mind, I thought, maybe tomorrow.

As a teenager with hormones surging, I discerned that the feeling of oneness was related to romance—what I experienced when sitting in the choir loft, supposedly paying attention to Mrs. Miller, our demanding director. Instead, I was sneaking looks with Danny, my heartthrob, who, after church, asked me to join his bowling league. I giggled and nodded yes, feeling that old tingle.

My diary from that year listed names of boys who took his place when he moved away. The names were in order of who was the current favorite. These were long lists. Much of my adolescent energy was spent plotting how to hold hands with one of them because that's a way I could come close to the special feeling. Occasionally, while cuddling in the rear seat of a school bus on the way to an out-of-town extracurricular activity, this rush of feeling would almost happen.

At seventeen, I enrolled as a senior in a newly consolidated high school and briefly wore the class ring of Wendell, the smartest boy in the class. We were elected the king and queen of the Valentine's Dance. I must not have recognized him as a potential soul mate because, as the year drew to a close, I began dating a man from another town, a charming man my mother adored. (She never understood and therefore didn't champion Wendell.) This one-year-older man introduced me to the joys of petting. Now the sensations of oneness I craved were the result of being touched by another. My strict rule was no sexual intercourse before marriage; I was deeply committed to this vow of chastity for the same reason I came to believe masturbation was wrong—a sense that someone would disapprove because of what I suspected were church rules.

I married that "charming man," my mother's choice for me, when I was eighteen, after a year of college. In retrospect, I realized this decision was fueled by a powerful desire for going all the way (the way we talked about sexual intercourse), and what I believed must be the most available gateway to the oneness feeling I was sure I needed.

The integration of sexual feelings with spiritual feelings was supposed to happen now that I had gotten married and put my energy into being a wife. The bond with a husband became *the* way I could merge with man and God. After all, religion declared married sex sacred. My husband made certain we were involved with organized religion no matter where we lived. After several years, he accepted a position in church administration for a large traditional Protestant church. His relationship with God was different from mine and our bond suffered for that and for many other reasons. Was I sad? Angry? Beaten down? Or unfulfilled? Disillusioned? Bitter? I don't know. I can see it in any of those ways, but I have lost many of my memories. I just know we divorced after thirty-three years. I was years into analysis before I began understanding what went wrong with our relationship and took responsibility for my part in it. As I said before, I needed too much, expected too much, and when I articulated my desires at that time, I did not realize they were unrealistic. I thought what I was asking for was possible.

After my divorce, having never lived alone, I hired a real estate agent I had known from the past, who sold lots of houses. I informed her I wanted a place where I could sleep upstairs and look out and see trees. She told me about a townhome she knew of that would be perfect for me but said it was not on the market yet. She was correct—I loved it. The contract specified I gained possession several months after our family home was sold. This meant I needed to move twice. I rented an apartment, but financially it made sense not to move into it until after the new year, which meant I would be homeless during the Christmas holidays.

An Episcopal priest friend, who was spending a year in Jerusalem, extended an invitation to visit her over the Christmas holidays. This offer was too good to pass up. I was single and could do what I wanted for Christmas, though my sister Nina was not happy with my choice. It was the first Christmas since Mom died and she would worry about me. My children all had plans, so I was not worried about them. The exoticness of traveling to Israel for Christmas thrilled me. Being single offered opportunities, I was discovering. Soon, my all-or-nothing thinking, thinking I did not recognize at the time as dysfunctional, kicked in and I imagined a fun-filled perfect adventure.

It was not the perfect trip I envisioned. When touring Jerusalem's streets on the sabbath when there was no one around, my friend walked fast and nagged at me to walk faster, not unlike interactions with my ex-husband. Why is everyone in such a hurry, I wondered. She chose to meditate twice a day in her small space, during which time I felt trapped trying to be quiet so I would not bother her. I decided she did not meditate correctly as she stretched out on her bed, just as if she was taking a nap, making herself comfortable with pillows--ironic as I look back, after my fussing about comfort with Denae.

It all changed one day while walking through the Old City streets, narrow as doorways, cows meshing with people, reminding me briefly of India.

Walking slowly towards the Wailing Wall—a part of the old temple in Jerusalem sometimes referred to as the Western Wall, I felt a pull forward, as if I were a part of something inescapable. I felt one with all Jews and all others who have congregated there through the centuries to pray. As I moved past the men's section to the place where the women gathered, I took a slow, measured breath.

I noticed first the singularity of each woman, the quiet, the intensity, the seriousness of devotion, the strong sense of purpose. And then my vision expanded, and I saw the color! Women with skins many colors attired in a rainbow of colors, moving, undulating, separate and yet together. I stood at the edge, watching, yearning for something I couldn't name. Then, my eyes settled on one woman in particular, bent over the purse she was using as a desk as she wrote on a small scrap of paper. When she finished writing, she wiped her eyes with the back of her hand and headed toward the wall where she found a tiny crack and tucked in her note. Then she straightened, looked back over the sea of women, making brief eye contact with me before she moved on, leaving space for another woman.

It was humbling to be in this place, a place I had never dreamed of being. A peace came over me, a sense of belonging here, an almost euphoric knowing that something nameless but important was happening. I savored the moment. But then, sensing the movement of other women forward, I hung back for a while, watching the drama unfold before me, letting it seep into my soul. In this holy place, tears welled in my eyes as I felt encircled by this sea of color and devotion, separate and yet connected, grounded and euphoric at the same time.

I tore off a blank page from my travel journal, found a pen and began writing. In this expanded space, I allowed into my rapidly beating heart, all the feelings of disappointment about the trip, followed by a wave of grief over my painful divorce.

Then I winced as I remembered the death of my mother just two months earlier—the woman whose womb had sheltered me and whose arms had encircled me for years. The pain and the grief washed through me into the words and when they were all written, my heart stilled, and in that quiet heart I knew there was room not only for disappointment and pain but also for love and joy. And I took a breath. A deep breath. Breathing in the pain and the joy and complexity of all the women gathered. And of Life. I stood on hallowed ground and moved into the crowd, taking my turn at the wall.

I wanted to place a wish in the wall like the women all seemed to be doing so I tore a corner off the page that I'd been writing on and wrote my wish for the future: "I pray for wisdom." That did not feel like enough, so my old self, the self that believed I needed someone outside myself to be complete, nudged to the front of my brain, and I, out of habit, listened and then added the phrase, "to recognize my soul mate." I carefully folded and refolded my wish and found a crack where I could insert it. As I stuffed the paper into this ancient wall, a sense of holiness overcame me again. And I knew everything would be okay. I turned and saw the sea of womanly color, and I savored it, pressing it into my memory, wanting it to encourage me up for the next stage of my life.

※

How could I have known then that the second part of my petition, the need for a soul mate, would be the easy one, though even that took much longer than I had hoped. But the first part of my prayer, the prayer for wisdom, turned out to be so elusive and so ambiguous, so transitory and so amorphous, that I almost gave up the quest.

Finally, I realized that I was looking in the wrong place. I was expecting it to be given to me from some source outside of myself—thus I searched for a man, I relied on books and ferreted out other people's opinions—when, in fact, what I needed was to develop my own inner wisdom, my knowing what was good for me, my acceptance of my limitations. The path I eventually chose to find that inner wisdom was an unusual one—Freudian psychoanalysis—a path that had been questioned by the modern theories of which I was a part. But this turned out to be a good path for me. However, "good" did not mean easy or quick. In fact, "good" turned out to be painful, sometimes to the point of despair.

―――

Before leaving the Holy Land, I hugged my friend at the airport and thanked her for hosting me. Silently, I wondered if she could see the difference in me.

Back in Iowa, I tried to cling to that feeling of oneness and holiness, but soon I was pulled into the chatty real estate agent's world. The agent informed me that the former owner of the property I was purchasing had confided that this property had been a healing home for her after her divorce. Certain that most of my healing had already occurred, I paid little attention to this information. I knew it was the right place for me.

On moving day, I stepped into the front door and immediately began deciding where all my furniture would be placed. I could not believe my luck in finding this home that had both all I needed and all I wanted.

The gas fireplace to bring me contact with the element of fire, always a spiritual experience. The cathedral ceilings. The windows that opened to fresh air. The ceiling fan in the living room. The kitchen with built-in appliances so much newer and nicer than I was used to. I walked slowly up the stairs, which I noted were a bit steeper than I remembered—a minor imperfection—and I fell in love with the loft at the top of the stairs. This would be where I would listen to music and watch movies; but more important, where I could sit, look out over the railing, and remember my experience at The Wailing Wall. There were two bedrooms and I pictured one of them with a wall of bookcases and my desk on the opposite wall. This room would be designated as the office. Then, I imagined how I could arrange the other bedroom for sleeping, so it would be in compliance with *feng shui* guidelines.

I went back downstairs and saw where my grandparents' classic round oak table would fill space in the dining room. Thinking about them reminded me of how they had given me rides to Sunday School before my parents were church-goers. Then I noticed the small deck outside the sliding glass doors. A very private space, I pictured how my lawn furniture would fit there to make a secluded hideaway for me and the new soul mate I was sure would be entering my life soon.

I thought of more information the real estate woman mentioned about the former owner and made predictions for my future based on that information. Since I knew that both the former owner and I were married to men employed by the church and both of us gave birth to three sons, I felt certain I would experience the same unfolding of events as she did. This would mean I would be married in three years and, as a result, be able to find in that union my longed-for sense of elation through union of sexual and spiritual feelings. I almost felt sad that I would have to move out of this wonderful sacred space in three years, I was so certain of my future.

༺❦༻

Little did I know it would be a decade before I would pass through a stage of preparation and healing and then be ready to find deeper integration from—of all things—Freudian psychoanalysis.

About this time of moving into my townhome, I discovered the words, *oceanic feeling* in the book, *The Self in Transformation* by Herbert Fingarette (Fingarette, 1963), words that described what I would eventually discover was my immature yearning for personal union, which was initially experienced in my mother's womb. I delighted in knowing I was not alone in wanting this feeling of oneness. By reading about it, I was reassured that others, too, wanted this feeling of being inseparable, of ecstasy. Someone else had named it and described it.

It was more than a decade before I questioned whether this oceanic feeling of oneness, of ineffable ecstasy, might not be a mature life goal. It took years of analysis to come to realize that what I wanted and thought I needed was something akin to an emotional and spiritual ongoing gratification through oneness with a man that was direct and complete. For years, it was a sacred calling, and I stubbornly refused to let it go.

It was only after years of living in my town home and years of analysis plus study that I came to understand more fully how Freud actually felt about the oceanic feeling. Freud called it: "regression to the primal unity with the mother."

Could it be that all these years I had been searching for something that would have been the opposite of my conscious goal, which was maturity and adult responsibility?

I yearned to find in Freud's writing some later understanding, some way of thinking about my heart's desire that did not mean I was regressing to the womb phase of pure pleasure. He had changed his mind about other things. Maybe he changed it about this.

Looking back, I wonder if I would have kept going to analysis if I had known that the goal was something opposite from what I thought I wanted and needed. Would I have stuck with a process that would lead me, not to oceanic oneness, but to the oneness I had discovered at the Wailing Wall.

12

I INVITED ROSANNE IN

My body had been trying to tell me something for months, but I denied a multitude of physical problems by focusing on research regarding the oceanic feeling. I was convinced that the deep personal work in psychoanalysis was to blame for these physical symptoms: that they were part of the transformational process, that they were psychosomatic in nature, and that they would go away on their own accord. I yearned to discover what Freud thought about the oceanic feeling, as I was becoming more curious about the type of man he was. All this resulted in my almost overlooking the physical malady responsible for my physical symptoms.

Denae was not giving me help to understand the symptoms I was having. Never mind that I did not officially ask her. I wanted to believe that she did not seem interested in my physical symptoms because I was not interested in discussing them with her. I convinced myself that she would not discuss them in the way I wanted them discussed.

I wanted face-to-face interaction about psychoanalysis with a person who did not treat me like a patient and who could help me understand the intricacies of psychoanalytic theory. The language of psychoanalysis was foreign to me and the sentence structures, convoluted. I needed an interpreter to learn more. It suddenly made perfect sense to me that I wanted to be a student of psychoanalysis as well as struggling along in treatment. This meant I needed a teacher.

My research online led me to long-distance learning classes offered by a psychoanalytic institute. The subject for the next online class—trauma from a psychoanalytic viewpoint—sounded interesting, so I enrolled. The instructor, Rosanne, introduced herself in an email with words and concepts that made me attracted to her immediately. Oh, this was going to be good, I thought! These were my kind of people. Perhaps I could merge with them, at least intellectually, providing me with at least part of the merging I had always desired.

When it was time for class, I opened the Zoom app and I saw the instructor Rosanne and immediately noted how her hair kept falling in her eyes. I wondered to myself if messy hair was a requirement for being an analyst. In the first class, Rosanne, the one other student and I introduced ourselves, and it was strange to say out loud that I had been in analysis for eight years. For the most part, I relished being able to share this without a sense of shame. In fact it was quite liberating.

I mentioned to Denae that I was taking a class from a psychoanalytic institute, though I did not focus on it and tried to keep it out of my mind when lying on her couch. I was reluctant to share the new information I was learning, as I feared she would disapprove and, unconsciously, I probably felt guilty for not telling her about it. Regardless of the reason, I did not want to deal with Denae's reactions to the class. I assumed from her comments in the past she believed my experience of analysis with her should be enough, but my need to know more and to be in control of something triumphed. At the time, I could not have understood the real reason for this choice, nor foreseen the ramifications of it.

As I had hoped, I received a lot of attention from Rosanne because the only other student (who lived in Central America) was often absent or late to sign on. I liked everything about this exotic instructor; her graceful maneuvers to arrange her expensive-looking wrap impressed me. Long hair twisted into an upsweep with strands falling in her eyes completed the picture on my computer screen. She described herself as multi-cultural and also as a pluralist. This was a new world. Because I believed that my body expressed my emotions through my physical symptoms, I was thrilled when I discovered Rosanne had a medical background and an interest in psychosomatic medicine.

According to Rosanne, French analysts are in the forefront of the psychosomatic field. I asked her for book recommendations on psychosomatics and it felt natural when she quickly gave me information about a 2010 book, *Psychosomatics Today* (Aisenstein, 2010). I was delighted with how Rosanne's response was so different from the one I received from Denae. I tried to keep the distinctions clear in my mind: Rosanne was my instructor, Denae was my analyst. They had different roles. They each were experts in their own ways. Once I had thought that through, rationalizing that I would not be going against Denae when I read books suggested by Roxanne, I ordered the book.

In class, I learned that, of all the things trauma takes away from us, the worst is our willingness (even our ability) to be vulnerable. This insight was recorded in my journal in big letters and circled, probably because I knew unconsciously that it was my lack of vulnerability that was making my progress in analysis slower than it might have been.

I learned that when we are wounded as small children, whether it is a physical or emotional wound, our self-protective response is to push the event and the pain of it out of our memories and into our unconscious, providing us a way to move forward. As is so often the case, a necessary self-protection at one stage of our lives can become counter-productive later, because this protective process, called repression, takes increasing amounts of energy, draining us of the ability to move forward. Later in life, it still has the power to keep us stuck in the effects of the original wound. This knowledge affirmed for me that Denae was on the right track in her work with me.

Rosanne zeroed in on my mumbling unintelligible words when I tried to define *trauma*. "Why are you having difficulty with that word?" she asked.

I froze. I did not know. My heart began to race. She waited, as if she knew already the answer and why it was so hard for me to speak about the word *trauma*. "Did something happen to you?" she asked.

Again, I froze. I wanted to respond in a deep and self-revelatory way. I wanted my self-knowledge to impress Rosanne. I wanted her to be proud of me and not be disappointed in my response. In effect, I would come to understand later, I wanted her to give me the affirmation I had received as a child and lost when siblings came along and diverted my mother's attention.

Primarily because of this one interaction, I kept thinking about Rosanne and wondering how I could keep her in my life after the class was over. I desperately did not want to lose contact with her. The relationship we established in the virtual world felt life-giving; so, I decided to hire her for supervision sessions even though her rate was unbelievably high. Her support made me feel special. She said she saw potential in me. She believed in me. She verbalized this. In other words, she gave me everything I thought I needed to be content and happy. She treated me almost as her peer.

Rosanne repeatedly said she did not want to interfere with the relationship I had with my analyst. During the months I worked with Rosanne, she was not always successful in fulfilling that intention. Mild criticism of my analyst and of her style slipped out occasionally. In retrospect, I realized that Rosanne should not have been undercutting my relationship with Denae. She did not have the same type of professional boundaries with her patients that Denae did.

My relationship with Rosanne created a conflict between Denae and me, though I did not consciously know this at the time.

This became clear when, months later, Denae and I discussed my foray into this psychoanalytic education, and she commented about Rosanne's interference. She was clear and to the point. She had felt the intrusion.

This disclosure from Denae surprised me. "That was a muddle," she said, as we talked about it, telling me enough so that I felt guilty, as if I had been, in a sense, caught in an infidelity. My mind flashed back to my first husband and the times he had been unfaithful to me, and I thought of him with a little more understanding and compassion.

13

My World Changes

Inner Voice 1: "I'm so upset. I do not know what is going to happen next. I want to know!"

Inner Voice 2: "Remember what you are learning in analysis and try not to be so reactive."

Inner Voice 1: "I'm going to crawl out of my skin if I don't do something."

Inner Voice 2: "Just calm down and think of what we can do. What are the options?"

Inner Voice 1: "I could take the last half of an Alprazolam tablet. It would not hurt anything. I was saving it for an emergency."

Inner Voice 2: "No, you don't want to do that. That's not a good idea."

Inner Voice 1: "Why not? People do it all the time! Why can't I? I'm going crazy!"

These voices in my head were the result of mounting anxiety and depression related to all the problems I was having with my body. I felt I could not contain my inner turmoil much longer. Barely legible, in spidery cramped handwriting like that of my elderly father, I had recorded what happened next. Once frantic voice #1 convinced more responsible voice #2 that this was no big deal, there seemed no alternative other than to open the bottle, shake the last half of a tablet out. Then just a simple swallow. Which I did. I was almost aware that I was making use of my favorite defense: rationalization. The pill was a minuscule. How could that possibly hurt me?

The chemical smidgen began to calm my sensitive system. Because of my rapid change in mood and my sudden capacity to again breathe deeply, it quickly became evident that my desperate feelings were rooted in anxiety—the type of anxiety these chemicals were made to soothe. The closing words of this scribbled confession: "What a difference!"

My words served as a justification for what had been a transgression. I thought I would be absolved by using religious concepts to rationalize my inability to tolerate anxiety and also to rationalize what felt like disobeying instructions for using my prescription.

For over seven years, I had rationed out thirty pills one-half by one-half. Only dire emergencies warranted a whole tablet. After that day, the 30 pills were gone. The prescription had long since expired.

As soon as anxiety dissipated, the guilt kicked in.

But then I quizzed myself, why am I making this such a big deal?

The inner answer was that I had made it a big deal based on warnings I received from my psychiatrist at the time he wrote the prescription on the addictive nature of these pills.

But the really big deal was my fear of addiction.

That fear was why I poured alcohol in potted plants at high school parties. There were substance abuse problems on both sides of my family tree, and I was fearful that—if I took one drink or one pill—I might turn out like my father's uncle who rented a room in a rundown hotel and was a disgrace to the family.

I resolved to confess my misdemeanor to Denae, but the next session was almost over before I spoke up. I adopted a vulnerable demeanor and shared fully the desperation of my anxiety and described how it had built up inside me. I disclosed the inner voices and my feelings of panic. I cried.

I assumed she would respond gently to my vulnerability, so when she said, "You know it only works for acute anxiety," I was surprised and dismayed.

I kept quiet. She continued: "It doesn't work for chronic anxiety."

My first thought was that finally she was saying that I had generalized anxiety disorder, but I was not sure, and I did not ask. Keeping things on the surface suddenly felt safer—a throwback response to my old self (the self that said, do not ask, do not probe; It is safer not to know).

Denae went on, "If you take this medication for chronic anxiety, it stops working and then it is hard to find the proper dosage."

The session came to a close and I left, relieved that she did not seem overly concerned. Maybe I did not have to worry so much about addiction. Besides, the pills were gone.

∽

The doctor I saw on the most regular basis was my osteopath. He worked in the clinic of a small university and specialized in manipulation, which is not a part of traditional Western medicine. His treatments kept my back, hips, and feet in alignment. When my body parts were in alignment, they were not as likely to cause pain.

I had been his patient for several years and was convinced that his help had kept me from becoming a crippled or hunched-over woman. His greeting at a regularly scheduled 2016 appointment surprised me:

"What is going on Nicky? You have such a wide gait when you walk."

As was usually the case, three students from the medical school associated with the clinic accompanied him. They all asked questions: "How long have you been having trouble walking?" "Have you fallen?" "When do you feel dizzy?"

I had trouble answering these questions. It felt as if I couldn't think, sort of like I felt when Rosanne asked me to define *trauma*. I, too, wondered what was wrong. I wanted to believe that my symptoms were the result of working on my posture. But everyone seemed so concerned and dismissed this as a possibility. I noticed my husband watching me closely.

The recommendation from the doctor was that I have a CAT scan, sooner rather than later. Everyone was obviously worried about me. I was a bit alarmed but sure they were overreacting. I thought I would be able handle this better if I just understood more. I needed to know what was causing it. Luckily, my husband was with me for this appointment, so when the doctor made it possible to have an emergency scan of my head and spine that same day, he drove me to the facility across town, which I never would have found. "Let's just see what happens," he advised

The osteopath received results of the CAT scan the next day, and my husband and I returned to hear the results. The scan indicated the ventricles in my brain were dilated and—most troubling of all—there were patches of brain atrophy. Of course, no one knew what caused any of these conditions, so a visit to a neurologist was recommended.

The office for the neurologist who had the first available opening for a new patient was located in one of the huge conglomerations of medical offices that I have tried hard to stay away from. The towering medical center was surrounded by multi-storied parking ramps. We drove around until we finally found a ramp without a blinking Full sign, and then drove for what seemed like miles more within the ramp before we found an empty place to park. I reached for my husband's arm as we made our way through a beautiful atrium, located and entered an elevator, pressed 3 and then, when the door opened, stepped out, confused as to whether to turn left or right. Along the way, we were sobered by how many suffering people we encountered.

"This way, Nicky," Wendell put his arm around my shoulder and guided me. I averted my eyes as we passed patient after patient who looked to be old beyond their years and in great pain. His arm tightened around my back, and suddenly I felt safe, as if we were floating down the corridor, as if I was the most important person in the world, as if this man would protect me from any harm, as if everything was going to be okay. I relaxed.

Then the nurse, mispronouncing my name, called me out of my womb-like state.

I grabbed the walker I had just begun needing to use, relieved to leave the waiting room. The first stop was the scale, which I wobbled onto by grabbing the rails, and I noted that I had lost one pound. When added to the three pounds I had lost just weeks ago, it pleased me—I'm always wanting to lose weight—but also frightened me. After stepping off the scale, I hiked up my jeans that were slipping down my hips. Well, I rationalized. At least I am not overweight.

Wendell and I entered the treatment room and the nurse put a thermometer in my ear briefly, and then curtly she said that she would ask me several questions. "It's a test," she said. I swallowed the saliva that had welled up in my mouth. She asked what year it was and what was the floor of the building we were on. I stuttered as I answered her questions, but I looked her straight in the eye, despite my nervousness. She left saying the doctor would be in soon.

Alone in the small room (that housed an examining table shoved up against the wall and three chairs), we sat and looked at outdated magazines and I read a brochure on Parkinson's disease. I blinked several times, thinking it was because my eyes did not want to take in such bad news: the symptoms of Parkinson's were similar to what I had been experiencing—namely difficulty walking—and it did not sound like patients got better. Tears threatened to spill, but I continued blinking and held them back.

The doctor finally came in. I sensed that English was not his first language, which softened my feelings toward him somewhat. I have never learned another language, so I admire people who speak more than one. I answered his questions and noted that he did not look at me very often; his eyes were glued to the computer screen where he was scrolling through (I assumed) my test results. Reluctantly, I looked at the charts and graphs he presented to me. I was just beginning to make sense of them when he cleared his throat and said: "It's possible that you have normal pressure hydrocephalus, which we call NPH. It might explain your symptoms."

I sat up straight and shook my head with confusion. I had never heard of this condition. How could a serious condition have the word "Normal" in its name?

The doctor spoke to my husband and explained the details of this condition as if I weren't in the room. They used medical language and words I wasn't familiar with. I barely listened as the neurologist revealed more comprehensive views of the scans to my husband on a bigger monitor, as I kept muttering to myself that I am not the kind of person who would have a serious malfunction like this.

Feeling a bit bored, I saw what looked like a dirty Kleenex under the examining table. Continuing to distract myself; I looked to my extreme left and saw how messy the counter was. I was unaware that someone observing me might think I was conducting an OSHA Inspection. I tried not to let my husband see how I was acting like a child; I didn't want him to think less of me. But, I did not want to pay attention to this bad news, so I used my old defense of denial.

"For one thing," I said to myself, "I would never have a condition with the word normal in it! I am unique." I felt a laugh coming on, or was it a sob?

Then Wendell rose and shook the doctor's hand, and we walked through the reception area and into the hallway maze, while clutching a list of tests the neurologist had ordered. On this list was an MRI of my brain and an MRI of my cervical spine.

The next week, I had another appointment with the neurologist, and by that time the results of the two MRIs had been sent to him. The doctor met with us briefly to inform us that a technician would be in shortly to administer a nerve conduction study. This test involved poking one needle (which was connected to a machine) into various places all over my body. I sat on the edge of a table, a white gown wrapped loosely around me, as the technician quickly poked the needle into my arms, legs and feet.

"Can you feel this?" she asked with each poke.

The painful test dragged on. Sometimes I did not know how to answer her questions about how the needles felt. After a while, they all felt the same. I felt overcome with a deep exhaustion.

When the nerve conduction study was over, we moved to a separate room off the consultation room, where there was a machine that tested my muscles—an electromyography. This test made me want to cry or scream or run out of the room. It was both time consuming and painful. The whole process the neurologist was putting me through was tiring. I already felt bad, and this was not helping. I missed my quiet home and my books. I did not know anyone around me, and no one knew me. It was all business to them. We were in and out of the offices fairly rapidly, though sometimes we had to wait in waiting rooms filled with suffering people (some slouched in wheelchairs), and people beside them with fear and sadness and vanishing hope etched into their faces.

Appointment after appointment. Week after week. Test after test. A new routine. Oh, these feelings. I was overwhelmed. Wanted to be home. Wanted things to be back to normal.

One notable afternoon, my husband brought our car to a halt by the automatic doors of the high-rise medical center where a sprightly male volunteer met us with a wheelchair. I could not believe it. I do not need a wheelchair. Or do I? But, I gratefully sank into it, because it was apparently ordered for me. They must know normal pressure hydrocephalus has a predictable progression, and that it would become (and was becoming) increasingly difficult for me to walk long distances.

The volunteer wheeled me into the atrium and, as he did so, confided to me how difficult his job was. He spoke with agitation of an incident he had endured with a nasty man. I was pleased to have an opportunity to make sympathetic counselor comments. I felt useful for a moment. He instructed me to remain seated in the wheelchair and left me in the plant-and-light-filled high-ceilinged atrium that we had walked through before. I breathed deeply and settled in the wheelchair, waiting for my husband to join me.

The atrium had a comfortable feel. I soaked up the simulated tropical atmosphere and enjoyed the clear sparkling light pouring through the overhead windows. I sat there, bundled up in my winter coat, woven multi-colored hat, and warm gloves, thinking about the botanical center, which always was warm allowing me to be able to take off these winter clothes. With no conscious effort, a feeling of ease and familiarity began to wash over me. Never mind that I was trapped in a wheelchair. For these few moments, I felt like a queen. I was in charge. I knew how to do this.

The feeling evaporated rapidly, and I may not have even remembered it were it not for the fact that I mentioned it in passing to my analyst. She wanted me to talk about the feeling and hinted that she saw it fraught with meaning.

The analyst and I mutually chewed on this filament of memory for weeks. It largely seemed a mystery to me, though the feeling of having everything under control was the element that I most recognized. As a kid, when I was not sick, I would set up a nurse's station in the living room, complete with pill bottles and note pads. I loved the feeling of being in charge of my patients, which at that time were my parents. Did I have those queenly types of feelings as a girl when I went to the doctor and then had to be hospitalized? Did I also feel in charge when I was ill? Was the queenly feeling related to my childhood defenses? Was it a way to rise above what was happening?

In addition to these questions, a concern that I tried not to bring to consciousness but one that remained in the back of my mind and made cameo appearances in the middle of the night, was the discovery—initially in the CAT scan findings and then reconfirmed by the brain MRI—of brain atrophy. Atrophy did not sound good, and I remember seeing dark parts on the screen that they said were the atrophied portions of my brain. I had looked away quickly. I was furious when the neurologist asked my husband if I had any memory loss and his reply was that I did forget things. I felt betrayed and was certain it was not me who forgot things, it was he!

There was no resolution as to why the atrophy was there or what it meant for my future. I wished I had never heard about the atrophy. All I really understood was the basic fact that the neurologist and the osteopath concurred that the results of the MRI confirmed the results of the CAT scan: there was an excess of cerebral spinal fluid in my brain. This was known because of my dilated ventricles. The doctors thought the excess fluid could be causing both my balance problems and the shuffling wide gait.

We learned of a procedure. It bothered me they did not call it what it was—surgery. The procedure's purpose was to insert a shunt in the brain. Tubing would be inserted from the brain leading to the abdomen. That would allow the excess cerebral spinal fluid to drain through the tubing to the abdomen. This controversial operation had a 40 percent success rate.

In order to see whether I would be a good candidate for the procedure, the neurologist suggested, first, a timed walk down his hallway. Next, an LP would be performed to remove a small amount of my spinal fluid. Finally, my walking time would be tested again after an hour. If my walking time shortened, it would suggest the procedure had a good chance of eliminating my symptoms.

Everyone kept talking about an LP. This is an example of the medical language that my husband understood, and I didn't. I finally asked, "What is an LP?" I lowered my head as if to pray when I heard that a *lumbar puncture* was another name for a spinal tap.

I continued to believe with all my heart that I did not have NPH. I wanted to believe it was not the type of thing that I would have. And if I did have it, the shunt thing would never in a million years work. My body was far too sensitive for a procedure like that. I knew it would not work. I would not be able to tolerate a foreign body in my system.

But there were no other options, so I made an appointment for the Dreaded Spinal Tap (that is what I called it). It sounded horrific to have a long needle inserted in my spine to slowly withdraw cerebral spinal fluid. I hated needles, so this was not something I wanted anything to do with. But it seemed to be the only way to know if surgery (which, by the way, I had already rejected) would help. I was **not** going under the knife.

Before the Dreaded Spinal Tap, I met with the neurologist to walk 25 feet down a hallway outside of the exam room while he timed me. I inspected my running shoes to make sure the laces were double knotted, and then I walked as fast as I could. I felt like a toddler learning to walk, with the doctor and my husband watching. The neurologist reported I made the distance in thirty seconds.

Then I journeyed to a different building for the LP. I felt shock when I arrived for the procedure (a word I would come to hate) and learned that during the LP, I would have to lie on my stomach. I do not know why I had not realized I would be on my belly, because I knew the needle was being inserted at the end of my spine on my back. I am always uncomfortable on my stomach because it makes my neck hurt. To be told I would have to lie on my belly and be still (because movement would interfere with the needle and cause injury) was not good news.

On my stomach, I felt more comfortable than I thought I would. I decided to breathe deeply. The nurse was comforting. I barely felt the needle. It was over and I felt so relieved. It was not as dreadful as I had feared. Alas, I was not thinking clearly at the time, or the outcome might have reassured me and reminded of something I'd learned in analysis: most of the disasters I feared turned out to be of no significance or they were helpful in some way.

After the LP, my husband drove me back to the neurologist's office for another timed walk. I was clocked walking the same hallway in fourteen seconds. There was lots of excitement because I had cut the time in half. I did not feel much different and I did not trust his timing. The neurologist had merely used his phone.

Because I was beginning to trust Denae a bit more, I wanted to process with her whether or not I would sign up for the surgery. But first I had to find a surgeon. The huge medical system that I was immersed in suddenly did not seem large enough. There was a wait before I could schedule an appointment with a surgeon. This gave me time to second-guess myself. Maybe I did have NPH. But why didn't they know what caused it? Why is the surgery referred to as a procedure? I really wanted answers.

It was December of 2016, and I was not getting what I wanted. I struggled with my body and felt confused and anxious. As I clunked my walker into a session with Denae, she handed me a sheet of paper. Being in the midst of high-tech invasive tests and doctor's appointments, and anxiety over how I would manage everything, I had forgotten something big: Denae would be out of the office for two weeks at the end of the year. She was always gone two weeks at the end of the year, but this year, of all the things I was facing, this felt the biggest shock of all.

My coping mechanisms kicked in and I began to hope that she would tell me where she was going and that she was sorry to leave me at such a critical time. I wanted her to assure me that she would be back. I wanted her to affirm that I was doing a good job of getting through all the MRIs and CAT scans. This situation was different, I thought. She would be different.

She did none of what I desperately thought I needed.

My journal entry reported, in penmanship that was difficult to decipher: "Hit rock bottom with Denae. I guess I have to have my own way. I fight her. Though something is not quite right in her interpretations, they may be close. I wonder if she's an oldest?"

14

CONVERSATIONS OF TRANSFORMATION

My sister Nina sends birthday cards extolling what a great sister I have been. I have never felt deserving of her kind words. She is different from me and not shy about showing me how different we are, sometimes in ways that irritate me. Nina is an extrovert and loves games with everyone, but especially with children. I am an introvert, and exhaustion visits me when playing games, especially with children. Nina wears cheerful primary colors, the brighter the better. I wear neutrals, shades of gray and black. Nina was reading *Ms.* magazine and talking about the evils of patriarchy when I was a young stay-at-home mother reading *Good Housekeeping* magazine. When Nina was into home decorating, I enrolled in college as an adult student. Nina's childhood nickname was Go-Baby, and she still is on the go. I like afternoon naps.

As an adult, I started to feel remorseful about how I had treated Nina throughout the years. Surprisingly to me, she was a frequent topic in my analytical sessions. When the analyst suggested that perhaps my feelings toward my sister were ones of jealousy, I felt affronted. My first thought was that Nina had never been a threat to me. She did not have thick hair like I did. Then I gulped, recognizing the superficiality of my measuring stick. So, I considered how she traveled the world when employed by an airline and worked side-by-side with her contractor husband to build a fabulous house; and I swallowed hard. I began to look at Nina with new eyes.

An incident from our childhood—one I would like to forget but that is safely tucked in my unconscious—made an appearance while I was lying on the analytical couch. I recalled yelling at Nina, using a harsh mean voice, chastising her for licking her lips. We were playing dress-up with our cousin, and it was time for them to try on lipstick. I was nice to our cousin when she licked her lips, but I yelled at my sister. I remembered being aware at the time of how unfair I was being, though I doubt that I apologized.

This seemingly random memory opened the door for me to the reality that I often had handled her intrusion into my life either by ignoring her or by taking my anger out on her.

Further proof of my blocking her out was my lack of memory of her birth. It was not just her I blocked out. I have no memory of the births of my other three siblings either. I denied being intruded upon by ignoring the discombobulated reality that I was living.

I did have fond memories of sitting around the kitchen table laughing at Nyla, the youngest, who made hilarious faces for us all. I remembered great times with Maxine and Lawrence, Mom and Dad's friends who had children the same ages as we siblings, and how much the adults would laugh and carry on when they were playing the card game Five Hundred. The two families met frequently in the summer at Pine Lake for picnics. When we took hikes, we walked by the places where the roads were covered with water. As cars drove through those spots drenching us, we would shriek with delight. We hiked the rocky hillside trails and usually lost our bearings which allowed us to experience the thrill of being lost. It was okay feeling lost with others nearby. One time when we thought we were lost for good and could not find a restroom, we laughed so hard we wet our pants. It is not that I do not remember my childhood; I just do not remember when my siblings were born.

Were the experiences related to my multiple siblings' births traumatic? Findings from recent trauma research suggest that sometimes memories are not formed when there is a traumatic event. If this is accurate, perhaps the trauma of having new siblings arriving every few years after my sixth birthday blocked me from forming memories and I must have simply risen above the negative feelings of jealousy and anger. This choice would have been highly approved of by my parents because neither of them sanctioned strong emotions, especially negative ones. And then, quite unconsciously of course, I became the perfect child so I could continue to receive the attention I was accustomed to, the attention I lost when Mom no longer was mine alone.

Of course, there was no way of knowing that it would be more effective to face and express the feelings of jealousy and loss than to pretend they weren't there. In hindsight, through analysis, I realized how I considered myself above such feelings. I was not the kind of person who was jealous or spiteful or even hurt or angry. I spent years with Denae denying these feelings, feelings I had not dealt with in childhood. In fact, feelings I had no idea existed.

When Nina's second marriage ended, she was sixty-three years old. As a single woman once again, she moved 80 miles from the fabulous house she and her contractor husband had built to start a new life. She chose a town where she knew no one, telling me she liked the energy of the place. Instead of getting a membership at the local recreation center she had been impressed with when she first drove through town, she joined the Center for Spiritual Living and said this was the first time in her life she belonged to a spiritual community that provided not only spiritual nurturance but many new friends.

When she first joined this group, she talked a lot about the power of positive thinking. Initially, her monologues were about the law of attraction, the idea that what you focused on was what you manifested. I thought it sounded like wishful thinking. I did not like it when she would scold me if I expressed anything remotely negative. For instance, if I made a chance remark that I was worried about catching the latest virus in town, she would launch a lecture:

"Don't talk that way—you will bring negativity into your life!"

I mostly ignored her; I rolled my eyes, even though (or perhaps especially because) we spoke on the phone and she could not see me. After several years of avoiding this subject (the power of positive thinking) and discussing Nina a few times during my analysis, I was curious to know if Nina still believed in the same way, so I asked her.

"Oh yes," she replied without hesitation, "I believe in positive thinking."

"So, how do you manage the negative parts of life?" I asked.

She was ready with an answer: "It is important to recognize the negative and feel the feelings that go with the negative. The feelings will shift and change. Then you go back to focusing on what you want because your thoughts bring those things into your life."

Her words surprised me; there was more depth than I expected. Our conversation was weird because I no longer felt like the big sister dispensing wisdom. I realized one reason for my irritation with her initial enthusiasm for the law of attraction and the power of positive thinking was that it was too close to my own way of thinking that Denae was trying to free me from.

When the power of positive thinking—the way of thinking my analyst labeled *being above it all*—ignores normal negative events, the result is likely to be the formation of the psychological defense known as *denial*. This was a defense with which I was very familiar and good at. I am indebted to my analyst for helping me look behind my defenses, especially denial, to begin to understand how reliance on positive thinking or glossing over pain and anger led to not being able to see what was right in front of my face.

In my first marriage, my focus on our avowed unbreakable bond blinded me to my husband's capacity to betray me—I missed signs that were in plain sight because of my inability to see what was right in front of my face.

As my analysis proceeded, I began allowing myself the chance to experience more negative feelings, the ones my analyst suggested were important to feel, though I still was not entirely convinced it was a good thing to do. Denial was a friend who was hard to abandon.

It helped when I remembered that writers I respected believed the power of positive thinking prescription was developed because of a reluctance to face reality. The fact that reality was not always easy to face made it even more challenging to do so. Beyond that, my mistaken notion (if I were good enough reality would reward me) was dying a slow, agonizing, miserable death.

Facing reality, without the sugar-coating of religious belief or the escape hatch of glossing over the negative, was making sense only after years of analysis. I held this new way of approaching all parts of the world cautiously. I knew that I did not know everything and would be learning how to do this until I died. Despite my fears, horrible things were not happening when I came down from my above-it-all position and felt painful feelings. I was learning to handle the complexity of feeling multiple ways about the same issue.

Several months after I began revising a draft of this book, I received an email from a writer friend who was working on his autobiography, commenting on how painful it was to describe—and therefore relive—the dark points in his life.

His words both surprised and impressed me. He was admitting that writing difficult things was painful. Why didn't I want to admit that reliving my dark times was painful? Why did I say tired and not painful? Sleepy and not angry? I was beginning to realize what my pattern was: to claim tiredness instead of feeling the emotion, to go to sleep instead of facing pain or anger.

During the opening moments of an analytical session, I spent several minutes bragging to Denae that it was my father's ice clips on my shoes that allowed me to arrive that day safely without falling. The first thing I remember her saying was: "I think that the praise you got in the oceanic world when you were alone with your parents was so total that when I don't give you that same kind of response, it's a BIG THING."

I reeled. Then I quickly changed the direction of my thinking. Those words were not up to her standards, I judged. A BIG THING. What a childish way of talking.

She was probably right—I did want praise to bolster me up, maybe more than was healthy, but her words sounded so silly. A BIG THING!:

"A BIG THING!" I mimicked her loudly, with a tone of sarcasm.

"You are ridiculing me," was her response.

I was horrified and humiliated. Was it true that I had ridiculed her?

She continued, "There is anger and rage behind that ridicule."

She offered this in such a reasonable tone of voice that I knew she had no doubts about her assessment. She continued: "What did you feel when you heard that tone in your voice?" she asked.

I whimpered, "I didn't know if it was really there or not. I hoped you would ignore it."

I knew in my heart I did not mean anything by it. I remembered thinking when I said it that it was a bit funny. It almost felt as if I was teasing her. I was sensing that I might get out of this unscathed, so I said with as much conviction as I could muster:

"I think there needs to be a place for teasing."

"Why do you think there is a need for teasing?"

Her response was unexpected yet made sense. It was a straightforward question that gave the impression she wanted to know. Why was there a need for teasing? I searched for an answer and then said tentatively: "Because my husband teases about everything and my marriage would be in trouble if there was no room for teasing,"

I offered that explanation as though it was a new idea because, in some ways, it was new to me. During my current eight-year marriage, I had noticed that Wendell teased a lot. There was no way of changing his pattern, though initially I tried. I was beginning to think I would not want to even if I could.

I muttered some more about the importance of making room for teasing and then remembered that I had wanted to discuss my developing feelings for her when I started the session, so I began to broach this subject by saying:

"I don't know whether the surgery to install a shunt or my sudden decision to give up my practice had the most influence on me starting to trust you more."

"You've seen me as omniscient."

"Yes, I have, except I kept fighting the notion. The surgery was a pivotal point in my learning that you were on my side. Sometimes I thought not having clients meant I didn't have to worry about what you thought about me as a therapist, and I would be able to relax more."

A pause and then she said softly and slowly:

"Maybe when you were working, your omniscience met my omniscience."

In the empty space after she offered those words, I began to sob. I felt her words in my belly. I felt them with my whole body. I continued to sob, but my tears slowed down as I shared these words:

"When I started working with you, I wasn't satisfied with doing family systems work any longer. I wanted to be a psychoanalyst. When I was working with clients and had questions, I wanted to ask you what to do. And when a client presented similar issues to mine, I felt uncomfortable dealing with them.

The tears continued but were lessening as the pain eased. I breathed deeply.

"You're feeling how your head hurt," she generously offered.

Surprised that she was talking about my physical problem, I responded, "Yes, having too much cerebral spinal fluid…" and then stopped abruptly. She was not only talking about my physical problem. She was using a metaphor to speak of the pressure I put on myself. I was speechless. This pause felt awkward. But, ignoring my blurt, she continued.

"You're convinced that if you feel regret, it will take over everything."

I nodded my head in agreement. I was surprised at her directness and clarity. I wanted to go on, but our time was up. I put on my ice clips and prepared to face the icy parking lot alone and yet not alone.

15

How Could That Be?

I feel as if I should apologize for this chapter because you as readers are undoubtedly getting impatient with Nicola's denseness. And then I remind myself, that when I set out to write this memoir, I wanted others to know what it felt like to be in analysis for a decade. How very difficult it is to change behavior and ways of thinking. Perhaps I am unusually dysfunctional. That of course is my fear. But in all my reading (and if you have gotten this far in the book you know that I have read extensively), I have found very few descriptions of how the analytical process unfolds, though I have read multiple times that the typical length of treatment varies from four to twenty years. You probably will not be surprised to hear that this comforts me.

So, perhaps being in Freudian analytical treatment for a decade is not unusual, but writing about how classical Freudian analysis works to help people get unstuck is the difficult, unusual part. Much of psychoanalysis consists of free association, the idea that speaking whatever comes to mind without worrying how one subject relates to another is the main way we discover what is in the unconscious. Freud advised analysands that they did not have to worry about losing their way when free associating, because the unconscious has its own internal logic and fundamental cohesion. It takes a long time to trust the logic and cohesion of the unconscious and I wonder if it is expecting too much of you as a reader to follow the twists and turns of my thinking. Perhaps it is inevitable that some chapters will seem repetitive and others understated. We all know that if one is mired deeply in the mud, it takes time to get out. So I hope this chapter will in some way be useful to you as I continue to use my experience as an example of how our human minds work. Of course, we will begin with my new heartthrob, Sigmund Freud.

Our first step will be learning about transference. Freud wrote that this is a defining issue of the psychoanalytic process, but he did not realize that it was when he began his investigation into how people's minds worked. Initially, when he saw that people responded to their analysts in the same way they related to their parents (an example of transference), he believed the response would be a problem and feared this tendency of the human mind would interfere with treatment. Freud soon realized, and I think this is part of his genius, that when people responded to their analysts in the same way they did to their parents it was a key to understanding the patients' inner lives.

That he had this insight so many years ago impresses me. Today this idea appears to most people to be common sense. However, even today we resist knowing that we are acting in ways and with motivations unknown to our conscious mind. We like to think we are in charge of our minds. Before Freud made this connection, humans did not recognize how often this tendency of humans to feel and see things that are not based in reality occurred.

According to Freud, transference is a normal part of personality function and is not in and of itself a sign of mental illness. Transference depends on the mental ability to deny that something happened and to transfer the feeling or feelings that were activated when the event happened onto someone else. For years I had helped my clients work through these issues. Women often had feelings and beliefs about their husbands that had more to do with their fathers than with their husbands, while men often treated their wives in the same way as they had treated their mothers.

My mother, in essence, had left me when I was six, though she did not die until she was 75 and I was 52. How could I have understood how deep my pain was over the loss of my special child status and how much I yearned to go back to that place of singularity? Yet, this was the stretch of time when I secured my place in my mother's mind and heart by hiding my feelings. It made me a good girl, after all, and what parent doesn't like a good girl. The analyst had tried and tried to elicit those feelings from me. Feelings that I thought would make me look foolish.

My rational mind had almost accepted how upsetting and traumatic it had been for my six-year-old self when my sister was born; I had lost my singular place in my mother's heart. It all made sense if I looked at the circumstances I had faced. But it was more difficult to come to grips with how that loss kept me stuck in a search for people who would see me as special, different, unique, above the rest. Stuck in a need for affirmation from everyone I knew.

Books affirmed me. My work affirmed me. Having my own therapy office affirmed me. I think this is one reason why, when this new health condition began, I did not want to think about giving up my precious professional office: ground floor, near the outside door; two sunny windows; three quiet rooms; art on the wall including my favorite print of color blocks by artist Mark Rothko, an artist I had studied as a docent. I created this nurturing space and was its occupant for ten years. Most people who visited me, whether clients or salespersons, commented favorably on the dramatic bright purple and red walls.

I did not want to admit to myself that closing my office would mean retirement. I had planned to work until 70 and, though I was then over 70, I was not ready to stop seeing clients. I loved my profession and wanted to work for many more years.

Talking to Denae about my professional life had always felt uncomfortable. Discussing with her closing the practice was even more uncomfortable. I remembered the few times we had discussed common-sense issues in the past, things like my health supplements, and she asked practical questions I did not want to slow down long enough to consider. I figured she might do that again, so I decided to make the decision on my own. I was stubborn, I admit. Since I could not control my symptoms, I think I wanted to control something.

Of course you need to close the office, an inner voice advised. Like a misguided immature teenager thinking suicide was their only solution, not realizing that things change as time goes on, I acted impulsively and without talking it over with anyone.

I would close the office by the end of January the next year.

It was late October when I declared my intention. My husband did not believe it possible to get everything done by then. His opinion made the adolescent in me more determined.

I knew I could do it.

I could make it happen.

Unconsciously, when I set the closing date, I must have known Denae would be out of town. She was always out of the office the week of Christmas and the week of New Year's, but I did not remember it consciously until she handed me the sheet. As I write this, I realize how much transference was still going on during that time. My growth psychologically was increasing, but not fast enough to outrun my complicated relationship with my body or my projection of my mother on the analyst. I knew that Mom might have told me what to do or she could have taken over and done the whole thing for me. So in a sense I was a teenager rebelling.

During the process of closing my practice, I did not go to my office. I did not want anyone to see me using a walker. I told myself that I did not want to see anyone because I wanted to avoid an awkward conversation but perhaps, unconsciously, I did not want anyone to see me in my changed condition.

I felt defective.

Defeated.

Humiliated.

And in that condition, I continued my almost daily trips to spend an analytical fifty-minute hour with Denae where I experienced the polarities of how sweet and how sour treatment could be. It was the last session before Denae left for Christmas break and she greeted me as usual. She ushered me into the consultation room as she always did. Today, I did not feel strong enough to get to the therapy couch. I plopped down on a leather couch and kept my walker close at hand. That meant we were face to face and I found looking at her weird. I felt vulnerable when our eyes met. I did not take off my coat or hat or gloves. It was freezing in her office (as it often was), and it seemed too much of a struggle to wrestle everything off for only fifty minutes and then have to put it all back on. I was very aware that this would be our last session for two weeks. I had trouble free-associating but somehow it did not seem to matter as much as it used to. I knew I was going to miss her, but I was reassured that she would be back. She had always come back. Our session ended with me looking at her for a beat longer than usual and whispering:

"I'm going to miss you."

She nodded. The gesture seemed full of kindness.

༄

I was correct in my assumption that she would come back. Right on schedule, Denae ushered me into the consultation room. I still sat on the leather couch. We picked up where we left off. I tried to disguise how glad I was to see her as I continued to silently seek out answers to the questions currently plaguing me

When I did speak, I did not articulate any of the important questions perplexing me. I mumbled about unimportant minutia. She still asked me what I made of whatever observation I shared and always, always, said, "Can you tell me more?" How could I tell her all that was on my mind?

Because it had always been difficult for me to admit my vulnerability, I hesitated when telling her that I still struggled to walk.

I was annoyed—no, I was much more than annoyed—with my body. I was furious. I had been in psychoanalytic treatment for years, conscious of caring for my whole self—body, mind, and spirit—and I did not understand how this NPH condition could be happening. While it was true that I felt more connected in my relationships (the most important part of my life) and felt more expansive in my interior landscape, an image I picked up in my reading to describe my mental state, still, I wanted to walk.

I lived with an assumption that time on the analytical couch would translate into good health, not illness. I never dreamed that, in January of 2017, I would be contacting a neurosurgeon to see if he could help me get back to normal. I did not want surgery. I knew I continued to sound like a toddler who would not quit stomping her feet, but I feared surgery. Besides, I did not believe surgery would work for me. I was certain my body would experience side effects from every drug forced upon me. Certain I would not survive surgery.

Also, I did not believe the diagnosis was a legitimate one. I thought it might be a hoax. I heard the neurologist remark to my husband that it was a controversial diagnosis when he thought I wasn't listening.

I did not want to mess around with a surgery based on a diagnosis that was deemed controversial and had only a 40 percent success rate. I was not going to be tricked into having surgery that probably wouldn't work. What was the point? I wondered if I might be ready to die. While I was not quite as obnoxious putting forth my resistance as I could have been, the negative chatter in my mind was far from quiet. It still wanted to be heard.

The session ended with nothing resolved.

At my next analytical session, after I mentioned the possibility of surgery and before I had a chance to articulate any of this, Denae asked a question that I thought contained an embedded judgment:

"Why wouldn't you try the surgery?"

I glared at her, livid at the implication in her question that it would make no sense to not give surgery a chance. Easy for her to say. It was not her head that was going to be cut into.

My inner toddler stomped her tiny feet: You can't make me have surgery. Leave me alone and let me die. And then added, dramatically, bring my sons home and I will say goodbye. I am ready to die.

But then I thought of Wendell. "Oh no, I can't leave Wendell. He already had a wife die.

How Could that Be?   199

And he's been so good to me and for me."

Then I tried to reassure myself, he would be okay, he would survive. Lots of women would want to marry him. He is a good catch. I will not be gone long, and casseroles will pile up on our doorstep. I guess technically, it will be his doorstep.

When I was being honest with myself, I knew that most of all I did not want to suffer. I did not want the pain of surgery. I knew it would be awful. This should not be happening. Of course, I did not say any of this out loud, but she kept talking:

"I think it's a no-brainer."

Oh my gosh! If I had been reclining on the couch, I would have jerked up and looked her in the eye. Since I was sitting up when she said this, and I did not have the courage to look directly at her, I grabbed my walker and banged it against the couch. I fumed! She had just said that the decision to have surgery was a no-brainer! She never said things like that! In fact, she had never said anything remotely close to words that would tell me what I should do or what she thought I should do.

I used to want her to tell me what to do, but not now! I think my MD husband is probably thinking and wishing the same thing—that

I would have the surgery—but he would never say it. I had been looking forward to her coming back from vacation for our sessions, but now I was not so sure. I got up, grabbed my walker and banged it, and then banged it again against the door when I left the session. Maybe I should crash down all the fabric screens that make the waiting room. I wanted out of there.

~

I carried this mood home and quickly surrounded myself with books. Snell's *Uncertainties, Mysteries, Doubts* (Snell R. , 2013), was again on top of the pile. A statement he made helped me slow down: "It must not be forgotten that the things one hears are for the most part things whose meaning is only recognized later on."

I asked myself, what meaning would I be able to discern when I gained distance from Denae's words? What did it mean when two of the smartest people I knew (Wendell and Denae) both believed I should have surgery?

I kept reading.

An obscure little phrase by Snell jumped out at me:

"Be alive to deadness."

This phrase seemed meant for me. He continued and now I read slowly the next few words of advice he gave to the analyst for whom the book was intended:

> Wander freely if carefully in the world of the person who comes, with all its sensations, sights, sounds, and smells, its lures, seductions, chance encounters, layers of experience, abjection, squalor and danger. (Snell, 2013)

Though he was talking to the analyst, it prompted me to think about my world with all its sensations and sights, its sounds and smells.... And I knew I wanted to live. And to enhance that living, I really wanted to be unstuck from all these old limitations. I had learned so much from analysis before the physical symptoms began. I wanted to get back on the road I had been traveling before these symptoms.

I left the book open but put it down for now. My compromised body felt energized despite the annoying symptoms; my cold hands slowly warmed. I sensed and felt the beginning of a relationship that I have wanted to experience with Denae since I began treatment. Could she have seen and felt the tension within me as I struggled, wrestling with what Freud named the death wish? Did she know that the death wish we all carry within was beginning to dominate my thinking?

16

Preparing to Prepare

Closing my practice was no longer taking most of my brain power. Instead, I tried to focus my hopeful attention on this: "I'm on the cancellation list for an appointment at the neurosurgeon's office."

My schedule book still recorded my four sessions a week with Denae, and I was thankful that there was something to write in the empty hourly spaces where clients' names used to be. I did not let myself think about not having an office any longer. It was painful, so I denied it. My symptoms continued: trouble walking, trouble making it to the bathroom on time, and feelings of dizziness. I still hated the walker. Maneuvering the walker and a purse was difficult, so I turned the walker into a sort of purse. The walker had a pocket, so I stored my Kleenex and Chapstick there. I was not driving, so when I went to a medical office, I added my Medicare and supplemental insurance cards to that pocket, plus my driver's license for identification.

My hand quivered as I grasped the doorknob when I arrived for a Monday afternoon session with Denae. I began to talk before we sat down. My speech felt garbled as my words spilled out telling Denae of the distress I felt at having to wait forever to meet with the neurosurgeon. I was semi-aware that I was rushing things and that this was a highly unusual way to begin a session, but I could not stop myself. She probably would not look upon this favorably. As I pulled my walker towards the couch where I was sitting, I noticed her face looked unusually stressed and sad. I immediately thought she must be getting tired of dealing with me. I reprimanded myself sternly for speaking before we even sat down. I was too much for her, I thought. I should have waited. Our habit was that I never spoke before we were seated, and we usually enjoyed a smidgen of silence. Or, I should say, I had not burst out like this for several months. But I felt so anxious that day.

When I was quiet for a few moments, she spoke, as if she was unaware of anything I had shared: "I need to cancel our appointment for Friday."

I found that I could hardly hear what she said. Was it that she would not be here Friday?

If so, I could not deal with it. How could she do that on such short notice? To me? She must be sick of working with me. Sick of me. The sound of her voice stopped my inner critic: "There has been a loss in my family, and I need to be out of town."

My self-criticism decreased a bit. This explained what I was seeing when the session began. She was grieving. It did not have anything to do with me. I felt for her, seeing the depth of her pain and yet she always stayed in her role as analyst so well that sometimes I wondered if she was heartless. But now I could see that she really did feel her feelings, which meant she knew what she was asking me to do was not easy. I reflected back on how I always told my clients that I would never ask them to do anything I would not do.

I began to collect my wits regarding what she had told me. I thought she said there was a loss in her family, that she needed to go out of town. She had never shared personal information with me since the very first time I met with her and she told me about her name. I felt honored by this revelation. Of course, I wanted to know whom she lost and where she was going, but I did not ask because I was certain that she would not tell me. At least she had given me enough information that I could feel compassion for her and not be angry she would not be there for the Friday session. The cancellation was not because she was fed up with me.

On that Friday when she was out of town, to calm myself and to help me to stop thinking about how long it would be before I met the neurosurgeon, I decided to read more of Sigmund Freud's work. It felt somehow appropriate to read from the founder of psychoanalysis when my Freudian analyst was not available. While reading a small pamphlet entitled *Psychical (Or Mental) Treatment* (Freud S., 2013), I did not read very far before my decision to read Freud was affirmed as a good idea. Here is the first sentence I copied into my notebook:

> "Illness originates from nothing other than a 'change in the action of the mind upon the body.'"

I desperately wanted to understand and believe that. If it was true, then I wanted to figure out how or what in my mind had changed to produce my debilitating symptoms.

While I was reading and pondering Freud, I noticed his use of the word: credulity. The definition: a tendency to be too ready to believe something is real or true.

I sometimes felt credulous in psychoanalytic sessions when I started to believe the analyst actually knew for certain that I was not expressing my feelings. How could she be so sure I was not? Especially when I would swear that I was expressing my feelings. But when I was courageous and went one layer further into my unconscious, many times I discovered that she was correct. There were feelings I was repressing. No one had ever seen me so clearly before, I suppose, because I had not shown myself in this way to anyone.

Freud wrote that the forces that created and maintained an illness were of a different order of strength, and that to give up an illness was a great sacrifice. I breathed deeply—perhaps in recognition? How weird to think that it would be a sacrifice to give up my illness, when getting rid of it was my strongest desire. I shut the book after I read the following sentence fragment: "powerful forces root illness in a patient's mind." I may be credulous, but if Freud's words were right, they gave me an opening for hope.

※

Even after my analyst returned to town from her bereavement absence, I kept reading and being enlightened by Freud. Reading Freud had a liberating effect on me. I started to imagine that the people I used to see in the coffee shop—the ones I envied, the ones who were concentrating—were also studying Freud. But not even

Freud could detract me entirely from the anxiety I felt about my body. Time passed slowly as I waited for the appointment with the surgeon.

༄

Weeks later, my husband helped me find the surgeon's office for my first consultation about the possibilility of surgery. I shook hands with the hands that might be cutting into my skull (though I did not immediately make that connection). I observed that the surgeon had a strange gait when he walked into the small examining room. It occurred to me that I may still have been projecting my own strange gait onto others, because it seemed the neurologist I had visited also had a strange way of walking. Were all my healthcare providers suffering from Normal Pressure Hydrocephalus?

The surgeon, who was an extra-large man, gruffly explained the surgery. He reported the success and failure statistics of the procedure with as much emotion as the announcers who read the boring farm market reports on the radio my dad listened to years ago. (I was always amazed at how intently Dad listened to the bean and corn prices when all I heard was a droning voice.) The surgeon declared it was totally our decision, that he would not try to convince us one way or the other. He suggested that we watch a PowerPoint slide presentation that would answer any questions. Then he quickly left the exam room, after indicating to us with a nod that I had passed whatever test the intake worker had mentioned that might prevent me from having the surgery.

This big brash neurosurgeon, almost in spite of himself, inspired me with confidence. I looked at my husband and we silently agreed to watch the slides, hoping they would give us whatever information we needed about the surgery. At the end, sobering clarity about what would happen filled the room; the procedure became real to us. The surgeon would cut into my skull, install a shunt in my brain, and then run a tube inside me, down to my abdomen, to drain the excess cerebral spinal fluid and allow it to be absorbed by my body's tissues. An additional incision in my belly would be required for the purpose of securing the tube. There was only one less-than-awful bit of news: the slides indicated they would not shave my entire head, as I had heard and feared (though I had always been curious how I would look bald, like the Buddhist nuns I admired).

The new sense of surgeon-inspired confidence firmly in place, despite the sobering facts, made it possible for me to authentically say yes to this operation. I looked at my husband again and we mutually agreed, at the exact same moment, to try the surgery. We saw the surgeon lumbering past the open door and respectfully called out to gain his attention and told him that we wanted to schedule the operation. He flashed us a look of surprise and said that most people took longer to decide. It surprised me that he seemed happy, after his sober no-nonsense presentation, but that was how I interpreted his sudden big smile. Quickly, he turned us over to his nursing staff, who obviously were familiar with the next steps of the process.

After conferring with the first group of nurses, I felt nearly euphoric at having this decision made, even if it was for a surgery, called a procedure, that I had not initially wanted. (I could not decide which felt better—to call it a surgery or a procedure—but I guessed it did not really matter.)My elation did not last long. I found out from the scheduling desk that it would be three weeks before the surgeon had an opening for the surgery. I deflated. Several weeks! I could not wait that long! I signed on to another list, this time for cancellations on the surgery schedule.

The interactions with my husband—as we met with the surgeon, watched the slides, made the decision, consulted with the nurses—gave me a warm sense of closeness with him. I did not yet associate the closeness I felt to the oceanic feeling I had always desired. This, like the free associations I had on the analytical couch, took time to develop, but would arrive eventually. We were one, but we were also two separate individuals. I was experiencing a new type of love.

During the following three weeks, I continued to see Denae for sessions. The initial upset feelings, which resulted from Denae's prompting me to have surgery, were soon followed by appreciation for her uncharacteristic encouragement of me to take an action. Multiple complex feelings rose up toward her. I figured she was not going to give me approval, so I was not certain what we could do in sessions to prepare me for surgery. This was because it was not yet clear to me that what I was really looking for and wanting was the close working relationship I remembered having with my mother. The times I was acting as Mom's assistant in the basement, while we gossiped and did laundry (over steaming double enamel-clad tubs that had a wringer in between) were highlights of my life.

I wanted to be working in tandem with Denae to prepare myself for the surgery once I had made the decision. But the sessions did not measure up to times I had had with Mom. Denae did not affirm me for the decision to go ahead with the surgery. I felt she had beat a hasty retreat to analytical silence, a silence that began to feel punishing. I remembered how my mom would not speak to me when she was angry, and how I struggled with the absence of her words.

In addition to the psychological part of the sessions being difficult, the physical part also remained problematic. I continued to need a walker to get to her office suite. I despised the walker, partly because needing to use it also meant that I had to use her creaky, scary elevator.

Then one day in her office building's bathroom, I glanced in the mirror, as I awkwardly turned around with the walker to open the door. There, before me in the mirror, stood my bulky, white-haired mother. She looked discouraged and downhearted. I suddenly remembered when I was helping Mom in a restroom when she was ill. She insisted on using only two squares of toilet paper. I did not know what to make of that. Was it true she did not feel worthy of more paper? Was it true that I did not feel worthy of good health?

One of the last sessions before surgery, I told Denae my legs hurt, and that I loved her and hated her. She wanted me to describe the pain, and to further describe my feelings. I felt so frustrated. I thought that was what I had just done—what I was doing! I did not know how to describe my feelings more. But I recognized she had a good point. The more I found out about the pain, the better I might be able to manage it. I kept repeating that I did not have words. Then suddenly, I said in a tiny high voice something like this:

"Mom didn't know how to manage my feelings of unhappiness about losing her sole attention. I did not know how to manage my feelings of loss and jealousy. Both of us kept smiling. We did not realize that expressing these feelings would lead to healing. We thought we shouldn't be feeling these things because everything was basically good."

As I squeaked out those words, I felt childish, while, at the same time, I felt like an adult. I was finally expressing my feelings. They were met with silence that now felt supportive. And, much to my surprise, when wheeling my walker out to the car, I had a lightness in my step. I did not grip the walker as tightly. My breathing was deeper. Lowering myself into the passenger seat and buckling up while Wendell took his place behind the wheel, I realized that, even though it was an intense session and I did not get any real answers to my questions, I felt better. I could visualize myself having the strength to live through the coming weeks.

17

NEEDING SUPPLEMENTS (TANGIBLE AND INTANGIBLE)

When the surgery, scheduled for February 28, 2017, was two weeks away, I found that I had two major worries.

1. How was I going to manage my anxiety without the use of herbal remedies?

2. Why were my analytical sessions with Denae reverting back to how they were during an earlier frustrating stage.

Both questions snuck into my mind frequently when I was awake and disturbed me when I tried to enter into the restorative sleep I knew I needed. The instructions I received from the surgeon's office indicated: two weeks prior to surgery the patient is to discontinue the use of any over-the-counter medications.

My anxiety, ramped up to accompany my ramped-up multiple physical symptoms, led me to use more over-the-counter supplements than usual: L-theanine (an amino acid recommended by my nurse practitioner); Calms Forte (a homeopathic remedy I'd taken off and on for years); and Emergency Trauma Solution or ETS, (developed by Perelandra Center for Nature Research). I didn't take all of them at the same time, or all of the time, but I switched around to get relief. I leaned on these supplements when I was feeling as though I wanted to crawl out of my skin. The very thought of being without these aids while preparing for surgery was, in itself, anxiety-producing.

I called the surgeon's office and talked to the nurse about Calms Forte, specifically. I told her I had spoken with the manufacturer and their representative said the tablets would not interfere with surgery. The company could not guarantee their product was 100% safe but, overall, they were reassuring. They generously offered to talk to the surgeon's office. I suggested this consultation possibility to the nurse, but she flatly rejected it. I asked her to consult directly with the surgeon. She said it would take time to consult with him.

The next day she contacted me with the news that the surgeon said he did not feel comfortable with me taking any medications.

None.

I was furious.

Then, without admitting this to anyone, I began to realize that this time I was not going to get my way. I could almost hear Denae saying, "You like to get what you want." Sometimes she used other words, but her meaning was clear. I continued to puzzle over how and why it was wrong to like getting what I wanted.

Deep down I toyed with the idea of what might happen if I really could not have my supplements. Could I make it without them? It was a tantalizing thought—both frightening and yet somewhat intriguing. Maybe I had made enough progress in my work with Denae that I would be okay. I consoled myself by thinking how things could be worse. Going without my supplements for two weeks was not as bad as having poison ivy blisters all over my body, I thought, the comparison bringing some comfort.

I wondered if maybe, just maybe, I could use meditation and deep breathing—bring consciousness to the situation—to get through the two weeks. Maybe I could, though it was hard to imagine.

Obsession with questions about supplements and also wondering why my sessions were so unsatisfying was not all-consuming; I had other things I wanted to explore while waiting for the surgery.

Because my devoted husband Wendell, a retired M.D., understood the medical system, he could explain what the doctors said (they usually talked fast and used unfamiliar words) and interpret results from lab tests. I wanted to think about how I could best express gratitude for all he was doing for me. I wanted to pay attention to his body language, so I would know when to give him a break from hearing and answering my ever-present questions. Because I saw him more than anyone else, I was also concerned that I might take my frustrations out on him, and I did not want to do that.

I, also, wanted to pay attention to my three sons, who were in various stages of arranging transportation to our home. Matt, the oldest, lives in Iowa, a long three-hour drive away, so we were hoping for good weather. His experience as a social worker caring for hospitalized elders would help him be with me. Formerly on the staff of a hospice, he knows about grief and is not frightened of emotions. He would ask questions that invited contemplation, and he would really want to know me as well as my answer. I predicted he would ask the following question (among others) with a seriousness conveyed by his voice tone and by direct eye contact:

"Mom, tell me what is most worrisome for you right now?"

Mark, the compassionate athletic middle son, had the very thoughtful idea of flying in from San Diego a few days before the surgery., so he could help me get through the days when I would be anxiously waiting. When I couldn't have my herbal remedies. I predicted he would say things I wanted to hear:

"Mom, you look beautiful!"

Mason, my artist youngest son, who shares my Buddhist leanings, and his wife, Lisbeth, a cardiac nurse, supported me with knowledge and love as we all speak a similar spiritual language. Mason and Lisbeth were arranging flights and lodging at an Airbnb for themselves, as (much to my dismay), Wendell and I would not have room for them all to stay with us. I predicted Mason would say:

"Mom, have you looked at the chapter on impermanence in Chagdud Tulku's book lately?"

I predicted Lisbeth would answer all my questions about body symptoms and fears with comforting knowledge from her years of experience working with patients. I could just hear her saying:

"Nicky, you are handling this so well."

You might think, after many years of analysis, I would have learned to name the short-comings of my children in the same way that I was learning to name my own, so I was surprised that my mind still gravitated to uncomplicated and idyllic words when describing them. I was hoping these descriptions would be the last holdout of my all-or-nothing thinking. I wanted my sons to be clothed in my mind's eye in multicolored fabric that honored their complexity.

In between thinking of these special relationships, I tried to find memoirs to read, particularly ones written with a psychoanalytic way of thinking about the issues I faced. I was in analysis, but I still had trouble knowing and describing what was happening to me both emotionally and physically. I needed to hear that others had similar psychoanalytic experiences before I could completely trust mine.

Denae had been of little help in lowering my anxiety level in ways I thought she should during this waiting time. When she mentioned during a session my "degree of wanting," I felt she was insinuating there was something excessive or wrong about it. I assumed she meant that I wanted too much support, too much love, too many experiences, too many things.

But when I looked up the word "wanting" in the dictionary, I found that it could also mean not good enough. Was that what she meant? I suspected not. Her tone of voice implied that she thought I was self-absorbed and greedy, wanting more. Or was I reading that into her tone?

I wondered, again, about the role of desire in my childhood. I suspected that I had needed to ask for very little during the first six years of my life. I wondered whether I had set that time as the ideal against which by comparison all other times came up wanting. My mother had been invested in keeping me happy, lavishing me with food and frosting, finding me beautiful clothes, taking time to play games with me, and, most especially, reading me book after book. In short, as a small child I wanted for nothing. Mom and I experienced and enjoyed a closeness that gave me a kind of oceanic oneness feeling of safety and warmth. The only request I made, according to family lore, happened when I joined my father in his request that I not be raised an only child. For reasons I can only speculate, it is likely that he did not want me to have the same fate he had for 18 years before his sister was born.

When a tiny infant sister arrived at our house, I wondered what to do with her.

Unaccustomed to having to ask for what I wanted, I did not know how to ask. The solution, (I figured out unconsciously, of course) was to be so good that people would give me what I wanted. Unfortunately for me, many times this strategy worked, so I was able to assume that people would give me what I needed and wanted without my having to ask or even admit to myself that I had needs. I am the oldest grandchild on both sides of the family and all my cousins looked up to me.

At large family gatherings, everyone knew: Nicky likes black olives! I was allowed to take as many as I wanted from the relish tray. I liked the pitted ones the best because I could eat them faster, but ones with the pits were good too. When my maternal grandfather returned from a trip visiting his relatives in California, he surprised me when, instead of the quarter he usually gave me, he said: "Nicky, Here's a gallon of black olives! You do not have to share with anyone if you don't want to. I bet your eyes will get even blacker if you eat all these!"

As a school-aged girl, I had to censor my biggest want of all: "Why can't things go back the way they were?"

I did not confess this want to anyone, scarcely allowing myself to know or feel it. Initially, I doubted my analyst when she suggested that this early loss was one I needed to recognize. However, I discovered through analysis, instead of asking for things that might ease my unhappiness (time alone with a parent, time alone, books, a horse), I devised ways of manipulating situations to obtain as many of those wants as possible.

While waiting the two weeks for my surgery, I began to wonder if one of the unconscious tactics I used as a child and then as a young adult was my suffering from respiratory illness. Psychosomatic theory would posit that our bodies are able to speak the language of our hearts more effectively than our minds. When my body did not produce an actual ailment, I was good at using a pleading look coupled with a verbal inflection to indicate that anyone in their right mind would see how deserving I was and give me what I wanted. My memory is that it usually worked. Those powerful ways of wanting or of getting what I wanted were undoubtedly what my analyst observed and experienced in her dealings with me.

While this presentation of me as a child may suggest I was unlikable, nothing could be further from the truth. I was a likable, a good girl when my wants were satisfied, and they usually were.

⁕

Before one of the sessions that took place during the two weeks waiting for surgery, my anxious mind returned to the same questions:

how I would live without herbal remedies and why were my analytical sessions so frustrating. I opened this particular session pleading my case in what felt, at the time, a very open and vulnerable attempt to verbalize feelings the analyst continued to urge me to express: "I won't be able to survive without using ETS. I need it to manage my anxiety. The surgeon's office said to discontinue all supplements two weeks before surgery. This worries me a lot!"

Usually indirect with her interpretations, that day Denae was direct:

"Have you spoken directly with the surgeon about this?"

Remembering my dealings with the office personnel and nurses I felt disgust at the whole medical system.

"No, I don't have access to the surgeon. I can only speak to the nurses."

"If you could speak to him, what would you say?"

I thought but did not express: I do not know why on earth you want me to speak to him about this. It is a hard and fast rule that is printed out in the handouts. What good would it do to speak to him? Besides, I am afraid, not only, of the big blustery surgeon but also of bucking the system, mostly because I would not be articulate enough.

These thoughts circled around and around my soon-to-be-invaded brain, but I said little. "You could explain to him the anxiety you deal with and see if he has any ideas. Surely, he has dealt with this before."

I received her response with mounting anger and frustration. "I know he wouldn't understand. He would say, 'Well I won't do your surgery then.'"

She countered: "How do you know that?"

Convinced she did not understand what I was going through, I wanted to stomp my feet and scream like a four-year-old, "I hate you."

But, Denae was not going to give up. I felt her implied judgment when she asked: "What is ETS?" It took me a few seconds to remember I had brought up the subject of ETS.

"It is a Perelandra product that I've used for several years. It stands for Emergency Trauma Solution."

I thought to myself; it calms me down!

But, I did not say that, either because I did not think fast enough, or because people tended to make jokes about it when they heard ETS contained brandy. My dentist, who had a great sense of humor, once brought me an airplane-size bottle of brandy, telling me that it would work better than the drops I used during our last appointment when he chiseled out an old filling. I smiled an inner smile at this memory, and then felt tears gathering behind my eyes. His death the previous year had been a shock I hadn't completely recovered from.

I brought myself back to the present moment. The mature part of me realized Denae was trying to empower me to speak for myself. But I did not want to be empowered at that moment, I wanted an ally. I wrote in my journal after the session that she could not make me talk to the surgeon. I took minor comfort in this adolescent rebellion.

I wondered if my assumptions about Denae were correct. Denae's interpretations were perhaps meant to be taken as helpful information, and I was taking them as disapproval. After thinking about this, my assumption that she was disapproving no longer felt rock solid. And, because of this, I felt less dysfunctional and a little less critical of her. Perhaps I was simply intimidated by her, fearful of how deep and painful our interactions could take me. That thought, on the one hand, gave me some comfort. But, on the other hand, could it be proof that I was making my world too simplistic in order to avoid engaging with the complexity of my unconscious.

I had had experience over the years with people who had tried to placate me, soothe me, flatter me, and defer to me. This was what Mom did, what my first husband did, what clients did. I was, also, used to people looking up to me. In the early years of my analysis, Denae began to help me recognize how dependent I was on the approval of others. It was true that I wanted her approval and that I slanted what I told her to highlight instances of maturity.

In a psychoanalytical session, there was no pandering or giving approval. The rules were different. I was invited to share all my deepest feelings in an intense and intimate relationship, yet most things the analyst said were in the form of interpretations that imposed frustrating boundaries on our relationship and felt unnatural. The analyst hid herself from me. I was not allowed to know anything about her, while at the same time she berated me for not expressing my feelings. Baring my soul, so to speak, I was finally coming to grips with the fact that the analytic relationship was not designed to be a normal relationship. Why had I not figured this out sooner?

༄༅

After years in analysis, I took a moment to take stock. My interior landscape—that space within where my thoughts resided—was enlarging, making room for new ways of thinking and ambiguous feelings, plus healthy self-understanding.

I was open, now, to initiating contact with interesting people and interacting with them with less anxiety. Because of my work in psychoanalysis, I had been able to move beyond an all or nothing way of thinking and I wasn't as judgmental. But now I was about to have surgery, during which a surgeon would shave off portions of my hair, cut into my skull, insert a tube into my body, and then make another incision into my belly so the tube could be secured. Fluid from my brain would then drain into my abdomen.

This was serious!

I wanted to rebel against the analyst and her method, the classical Freudian method. Because of my situation of facing surgery, I wanted nurturance and care in the way I had always received it during circumstances like this.

Never mind that care in that form in the past had kept me dependent.

I did not want to be reminded of my strong need to be cared for and comforted—I didn't care about knowing the ways I got in my own way.

The analyst would, at a later date, garner my appreciation for taking the heat, thereby protecting my husband and children from being the targets of my angst. But not now.

I may not have wanted to be at the hospital at 6 a.m., but there we were, all shivering in unseasonably cold weather as Wendell, Mason, and Lisbeth escorted me from the car to the surgical wing.

Mark had departed early for San Diego, having done his job of keeping my mind off surgery by coaching me on the fine points of exercises on my TRX Suspension Training system. I liked that it was advertised as using your body as your machine and I felt strong using it.

Matt would be driving to town to be with me later.

Mason and Lisbeth were with me. Both were physically demonstrative, and I soaked up all their hugs and encouraging words.

Wendell, in the background, remained attentive and I remained grateful for his presence.

I could feel myself beginning to bask in being the center of attention, as I was when pneumonia sent me to the hospital as a child.

The anesthesia was administered.

Worry faded. Thoughts drifted away.

18

I WAKE UP?

I woke up. At least, I thought I was awake

Of course, I did not have my glasses yet and everything had a sparkly effect, courtesy of my cataracts. I did not have my watch and could not make out the time on the wall clock. I wondered how long I was under the knife. And how long I would be in this room.

As if in answer to my questions, I was wheeled to the recovery room. On this journey, all I saw were blurry florescent lights surrounded by ceiling tiles. The tiles reminded me of the ones I scrutinized while lying on Denae's analytical couch. The nurses pushed the bed too rapidly for me to study and interact with these tiles, which felt like opportunity lost. But that was okay, I had a question that desperately needed an answer.

"Did everything turn out okay?"

Wendell held my ringless hand and assured me the surgeon's report was good.

Relief flooded through me, accompanied by an image of the Sumerian goddess Inanna, the goddess of sex, war, justice, and political power. On her way to the underworld, Inanna was forced to forever surrender one of her treasures at each gate. Remembering being stripped of both my wedding ring and the ring I had worn on my right hand every day since 1994, a ring given to me on my first trip to India, I was grateful that my descent had not been as dramatic as Inanna's.

Leaving the recovery area, I presumed I was enroute to my private hospital room. Instead, I was taken to a huge room with fabric screens separating the beds—a holding tank for people who were waiting for their rooms. The screens circling my bed reminded me of Denae's office screens. I glanced around me—screens to my left, screens to my right, and screens right in front of me. I began to fade, transported to Denae's waiting room.

"There isn't a room available," the nurse told my husband. Her voice intruded on my reverie.

I continued to fade in and out of awareness. We kept asking, "When will the room be available?" The nurses profeseds ignorance.

We waited and waited. Only my husband was allowed in this space with me. I knew that my family members were in the building; I yearned to see them.

Someone handed me a puffy plastic bag with my name on it. Initially, when I peeked inside, I gasped. The bag was bulging with white hair! My mother's hair! When had I turned into my mother? How much hair had they shaved off for the incision? I had been told that, in order to see where to insert the shunt into my brain and to clean the area for the incision, some hair would be shaved. This bag looked as if it contained my entire head of hair. I fretted about what hairstyle I would have to adopt to camouflage such a big bald spot.

I had something new in my brain, I mused. It felt odd to say, "I had brain surgery." As my psychoanalytic ability to free associate kicked in, I admonished myself not to focus on hair as I had in the past—obsessing about whether my bangs were too heavy or too short or if the proportions of a new style fit my face. My hairdresser, a saint who knew how fussy I can be about my hair, would know what style to use to cover the bald spot. I did not have to worry so much about what my hair looked like anymore, I realized. There were more important issues. In the past, I had thought of my hair as looking either good or awful. Now, I realizes, no one besides me much cares.

So, I forgot about the sack of hair as well as the remaining hair on my head and focused on my accessorized-with-a-shunt brain. When I said the word brain to myself, a poignant and all-consuming free association appeared: brain group. Soon I was diving deep into fond but confusing memories of a long-standing salon-type group that I gave birth to over 20 years ago.

Questions about my relationship with the group popped up rapidly. Why on earth was I afraid to disclose to them that I was in analysis?

One day I was late getting to my office where the meetings were held, and they were waiting in the hallway outside my doorway.

"Here, let me unlock the door. Sorry I'm late."

They assured me that they had only been there for a few minutes.

"Sorry," I mumbled again. I hesitated, thinking this would be a perfect time to tell them I was in analysis, and that I had just had a tough session, after which I had rushed to the restroom to get control of my emotions and wipe off smeared mascara. But what came out of my mouth was: "The traffic was bad."

One member of the group did not believe in the unconscious, and, entranced by the new brain research, had suggested we study the book, *The Neuroscience of Psychotherapy*. We had all agreed to read and discuss the first chapter of the book for this session. During my reading, I was extremely relieved to see Freud quoted—sentences that stated participation in analysis required a healthy dose of ego strength or, otherwise, the stress of analysis would send people over the edge.

I had savored this sentence when I had read it and then almost disclosed I was in analytic treatment. Almost.

I had wanted to believe Freud. Needed to believe it.

I could not be in analysis if not fairly healthy!

༄

Lying in the hospital bed just out of surgery, with little control over where my mind drifted, something inside me relaxed. Some tension eased. Some gentle acceptance of myself crept toward consciousness.

Continuing to wake up, I turned my head to rest on my right side, the side on which I usually slept curled in the fetal position. The incision on the right side was very tender and painful.

I could not lie on it comfortably. I thought of how Denae had commented on how insistent I was on comfort and decided this discomfort was tolerable. Of course, it was sore. Pain is a part of life. Thankfully, I no longer expected my thinking would or could banish suffering.

We left the holding tank with the familiar-looking screens and were finally escorted to a long narrow awkward hospital room that would be mine for the night. The nurse said I could use the restroom, so, walker in hand, I made my way to the toilet. While there, someone from the hospital brought a plant with an apology note for the room not being available sooner. I liked the plant almost enough to forget my irritation about the room delay. Something green brought life to this sterile environment.

While I was making my way back to the bed, Mason and Lisbeth arrived. "Your feet are moving so much better," Lisbeth said, accessing the skills she developed during her life as a cardiac nurse. "You are not shuffling!"

Her words felt like approval and admiration. I was pleased with her and with myself. Staying in her nurse role, she remarked

"Your vitals are good!"

I smiled.

I was given a plastic device and told to blow into it hard enough to make a bead move up a tube. Success would indicate my lungs were clear. It was hard to move the bead up the tube and nobody in the room was sure how many times I needed to accomplish this feat. I decided not to fret about it and set the device down.

The hospital nurse wanted me to walk down the hall using the walker. After an ordeal getting my shoes on, I made it all the way down two hallways and back. My husband, son, Lisbeth and two nurses, congratulated me with what appeared to be excessive enthusiasm on my walking. They said how much better my gait was and kept commenting, "You're not shuffling."

In truth, my walking did not feel all that much different. Were they being patronizing?

Everyone knows how to walk, I thought.

I did not feel very balanced and I was lightheaded.

The nurse instructed me on how to use the walker in the future so that it would not hurt my back. Her instructions made my relationship with the walker more complicated. I was not sure I understood what she meant, and she spoke so fast. I was trying to be as happy as my family all seemed to be, but it was difficult.

My visitors bundled up to leave and gave me hugs and kisses and good wishes. A surprising calm descended once they were gone. The nurse came in to prepare me for bed, and I began to free associate about my affinity for hospitals. I had learned that the way we respond to places and people does not change much as we grow up, unless we undergo some intervention like psychoanalysis; so by reverse logic, we can imagine quite accurately how we would have responded as a child.

I closed my eyes and found the self I used to be, remembering how bumpy and dusty the gravel road from our farm to the doctor's office in town was. I was seven years old and alone in the car with my Mom. She was driving. I pictured the two babies that had invaded our home, cute but bothersome, who were now staying with grandma so Mom could take me to the doctor. Since there was not much time for Mom and me alone anymore, I yearned to talk to her like we used to talk. My voice was difficult to rally because my deep chest cough kept interfering. Finally, I was able to ask her, "Mom, do you think I will have to stay in the hospital tonight?"

Inwardly, I remember wishing the doctor would say, like he did three years previously, "Go directly from this office to the hospital. Do not go home." At that time, I did not want Mom to leave me, but this time I thought it would be a relief to go to the hospital. I knew people would bring me books and treat me as special. But I also knew that my going to the hospital would cause Mom a lot of work and that Dad would worry about the money, so I pretended to Mom that I was worried about going to the hospital. To my parents relief, I did not have spend the night in the hospital.

When this free association was interrupted, I gave to my younger self the wisdom I have learned in analysis: You did the best you could. You do not need to be sick to get attention. I swallowed and repeated to my grown self with head wrapped in a bandage, "You do not need to be sick to get attention."

Lying in the post-surgery bed, I understood this desire to be hospitalized, this intense wish that previously had puzzled me. It was a young girl's way of dealing with loss—the loss of being held as singularly special, of floating in a world where pain brought attention, of being embraced and assured that attention would always be available. And then having it all end when the house began filling up with other children.

I saw in my mind's eye how that young girl protected herself by believing that she must have done something wrong and that was why her mother, now, paid so much attention to her siblings. In this way she had some sense of control. If she had caused the problem, she could fix it. All she had to do was be good enough and nice enough and helpful enough and loving enough, and her mother's attention would return to her. She also tried to concentrate on the good times when she enjoyed reading in her room and fantasizing about having a horse. But unconsciously this younger self must have still believed that she needed and deserved the singularity of attention and love she had had and missed. So she turned to others—teachers, coaches, friends, boyfriends—to receive the singularity of attention she needed, attention that felt wonderfully familiar. By doing this, she could get along just fine.

Lying in that hospital bed, I felt a rush of understanding and love for my past self. I understood her need to try too hard, to need too much. I could love her without being her anymore. So, I promised myself that I would work at no longer blaming myself when things were disappointing and did not turn out as I planned. And that I would ask for time alone. And continue to practice the vulnerability I was learning about in analysis. This last one was the hardest.

When I found out the next morning that one night was all I needed in the hospital, I was elated. I felt weak but was beginning to feel cheered by everyone saying I was walking differently and that I looked healthy.

My vitals, as Lisbeth kept telling me, were good. I'd never given my body credit for maintaining my temperature and pulse rate and blood pressure. Lying in that hospital bed, I thanked my body for maintaining itself and vowed to be more appreciative in the future.

I bundled up and was pushed in a wheelchair to the front entrance to meet my husband and Mason and Lisbeth for my ride home.

Once home, I slid into fretting about the symptoms I continued to have, they were not completely gone.

Why couldn't I walk normally yet?

Would I have to wear what I reluctantly called adult diapers forever?

What was interfering with my sense of balance?

Was my thinking the night before, when I had reached a state of serenity about my past, just me being wacky from the anesthesia?

"Time for you to get up and walk," Wendell broke into my self-interrogation. I needed to focus on walking. The surgeon told my husband it was important for him to get me to walk every day. So I pledged to Wendell that I was going to practice walking every day and go to physical therapy as instructed. I wanted to be able to walk boldly back into life, and then through the rest of my life.

And I pledged to myself that I would try to listen to my analyst; maybe not read quite so many books. I'd focus on our work together. Maybe I would be able to see better how far I had come since the night I ran off the road and got stuck in the mud.

Commitment to goals was important, but more important was my desire to trust the layout of my new inner landscape. A decade of psychoanalysis had slowly shaped me into a person who could both enjoy greater health and experience compassion for myself and others. I wanted to live my life—not in a rush for completion or denial or running away from suffering—but listening to what is. As I scanned my mind, I took a deep contented breath. Could I be ready for my analysis to end?

19

ONWARD

∞

The day began with an interruption to my daily meditation preparations, an interruption that unsettled me enough that, afterwards, I found it hard to sit focused on my breathing for even ten minutes. A former client had died. A woman younger than me. Staring out the window, I noticed dark clouds rolling across the sky, signaling a storm on its way.

Later that day, driving through biting rain to meet with my analyst, I noticed the rain was trying to melt the enormous piles of dirty winter snow. The showers seemed a harbinger of spring, but with temperatures barely above freezing, the snow was not melting. Nature seemed reluctant to end winter.

Death and coincidence were on my mind. Also on my mind was an emerging concern about how to complete the writing of my memoir while simultaneously continuing analysis. And always present subliminally was the question of how and when to terminate analysis.

My mind was buzzing. I stretched out on the couch.

I began the session with short bullet-like sentences: "A former client—who felt like a friend—died. I learned this from another former client. Was this a boundary-crossing violation?" And then, hardly pausing to breathe, I blurted out, "I am suspicious of my latest insight that I don't have to end analysis in order to wrap up the memoir."

I could hear urgency in my voice. It felt essential that this information be verbalized before I proceeded to the daunting task of free association. If I had stopped to think, I would have remembered that dumping information at the beginning of a session in this manner had never generated a meaningful session. But occasionally, I did it anyway.

The depth work I craved would begin when I slowed down, changed my level of consciousness, let silence settle into the room, and listened for free associations that might sneak past my internal censor. Fully aware that a successful free association could occur only when I expressed whatever appeared from the unconscious without hesitation, I nevertheless frequently failed to shut down my inner editor, breaking the rule Freud had declared was a foundational principle of psychoanalysis—say everything and anything that comes to mind. Still, I had come to trust Denae, and when I finally finished blurting out the faux free associations of my planned thoughts, I fell silent.

Denae broke the silence, "A friend dying, ending your memoir, terminating analysis. It seems they are all intermingled."

I smiled to myself, pleased she made an understandable interpretation.

Then mental clouds rolled in making my pleasure short-lived. I wanted to know what this intermingling meant, even though I had been learning that this was not the way analysis worked. I wanted to trust my unconscious and listen. Yes, I knew that closure was what all of these had in common, but where did that leave me? What was I going to do? What was she trying to tell me?

I waited.

I thought.

I tried to feel.

It crossed my mind that I had always had a fascination with the grief process. Maybe that was what this intermingling was about. Grief.

I waited and she eventually spoke again: "Does the decision on how to end analysis and end your memoir seem similar to your decision to close your practice?"

Her question caught me by surprise, though I would have thought after all these years I would expect the unexpected from her. I did not quite understand what she was asking, but I tried to stay with it.

I remembered all the years of analysis when, if her question nudged me toward some painful place, I simply moved from an emotional response to a thinking response, questioning the question, then questioning the questioner, either that or quickly moving on to other thoughts, other memories, or other situations.

Finally, I realized the pattern I had developed of fighting her by ignoring what I did not want to hear. Then, she offered, in a gesture akin to mercy:

"You didn't like what I said, so you blocked it out."

For many years, I would have sworn that I was open to others and their opinions. After years of analysis, I now questioned whether or not I was as open to others and their opinions as I had thought. New behavior happened in this session when I accepted her interpretation—I didn't avoid it. I considered how I had closed my practice.

Then, latching onto one of my favorite defenses—intellectualizing, I dropped the name of an author and I told Denae how this author had written that the infant was quick to separate the world into good or bad; that, when the mother's breast was there, it was a good breast and when it was not there, it turned into a bad breast.

No comment.

I blundered on even further to explain my association: "I probably felt interest in this example because I still separate things into good and bad categories. You know, my all-or-nothing thinking."

No comment.

I continued, my voice lowered and trembly:

"I didn't even visit my beautiful, colorful office once I made the decision to close it. I didn't want anyone to see me using a walker."

Finally, she responded: "Why didn't you want people to see you using a walker?"

I tried to answer the question but found that I really did not know what my horror of being seen was about. Because that was how it felt—horrible. I began feeling into the question—remembering those times when it felt my body was betraying me, remembering the pain, the awkwardness, the fear, and my shame. While I was drawing up memories, she murmured: "Our time is up."

As I rose from the couch and headed for the door, I knew I was on the edge of something important, some breakthrough, and I berated myself for wasting so much time at the beginning of the session. But then, as I walked down the hall, I realized how stuck I was in this particular critical response, spinning my wheels, digging myself deeper and deeper into my frustration. And I had been doing this since the beginning when I left sessions: berating myself either for wasting time on unimportant subjects or for staying on the surface of things and pretending the surface was important; or I berated her for some failure to understand me.

This time I stopped, took a deep breath, and propped open the outside door with my foot so I could raise my umbrella. I noticed, as I headed for the car, that the rain (that had been pouring down when I arrived) had let up, the excess water had already drained off the streets after washing them clean of dirt and hidden ice that could have sent me skidding toward the ditch. In fact, streaks of light were breaking through the clouds.

I got in the car and started laughing. Another typical session. Another hour in which it seemed nothing was accomplished. And yet here I was, feeling lighter, somehow, ready to go home to my husband who loves me just as I am, ready to love him in return as well as I can, ready to live out another day of my perfectly imperfect life. I felt a rush of contentment, even joy, emotions that had mostly been inaccessible to me before analysis, but now came and went, as did other feelings, like grief and anger.

Was it that simple? Had it been that obvious all along? Had I just needed to redefine my goal? My goal, now, was not to reach some ideal of contentment, some perfect environment like the one I had before I was born and for too long afterwards. Rather, I wanted to have access to all my emotions and the ability to make choices about my behavior based on them.

I thought back on the pace of my life at the time I went into analysis and compared it to the pace now. At first blush, it had hardly changed. Though I was no longer meeting with clients twenty hours a week, I was still active, still reading and exploring various spiritualities, still tending to my body, still enjoying time with my husband and family and friends. But somehow it felt different, as if my activities were less an attempt to escape that nagging anxiety that I had done something wrong or that I was missing something, something important. Now

I was more often than not propelled by gratitude for all I have, for the wonder of life itself.

Sitting there in the car, I realized that I trusted the work I had done, trusted it enough to know that it will never be complete, trusted it enough to see my past self with compassion; to experience my present self with loving kindness for the day, even a day when I regress; and to think about the future with curiosity. I can trust that what has been will lead to a lifetime of what is—living, not stuck in patterns from the past, but open to the experiences of the day and propelled forward with a new-found energy.

I turn on the engine, hear the motor hum, shift into drive and head home.

Closing Scene

I reluctantly click to end the zoom celebration with my editor and then take a deep breath. We were celebrating getting our first proof copy and actually seeing my words in print! I cradle the book to my heart for a moment and then look at it again, savoring the cover's dark red background, the symbolic gold swath connecting the conscious and unconscious and the regal orange letters that highlight the swath. I think about the process, both for the book and for the cover. I knew what I wanted for the book, but did not have the skill to write it; and I knew how I wanted the cover to look like but did not have the design skills to make it happen. In both cases, I had the wisdom to get help and the strength to hold onto my vision. I grin to myself that I might be describing intersubjectivity—*the magic word I kept trying to manifest with Denae.*

I flip through the pages, seeing word follow word flowing through the book describing my psychoanalytic treatment. I glance up at the portrait of

Freud above my monitor and remember how disturbed I felt when I read that he told patients the goal of analysis was not to solve all the problems of life—only the ones they had made for themselves. Who makes problems for themselves? I had wondered.

Now I understand his words.

The process of terminating my analysis, set in motion a year ago, is nearing completion. The sadness over ending my relationship with my analyst feels like the grieving that washed over me when I faced my mother's death. And at the same time the process of finishing this book, which means letting go of my editor—the woman who believed in the value and power of my words and brought them to full term, who midwifed my book through the birth canal, and who offered support well beyond the tweaking of words—leaves me awash in feelings of pure, raw grief.

For a moment, I wonder if I can bear so much pain. So much loss.

The memory of how I handled situations like this a decade ago appeares as a free association: before analysis I would have denied the pain, stuffed the memories, and decided I was being ridiculous for feeling so much. By repressing such feelings, I was able to rise above it all.

Briefly, I contemplate how easy it would be to escape this deep sadness and loss. What would it matter, just this once, if I retrieved one of my old defenses?

I sit back in my chair and, out of the corner of my eye, see the washing machine and recall Denae connecting my desire to do laundry to my desire to clean up emotional feelings. I look back at my desk. I know I could spend days cleaning this desk piled with books and papers to take my mind off pesky emotions.

Then, I would feel the satisfaction of accomplishing something. And perhaps the emotions would be gone—or at least manageable by the time I finished.

It's tempting, but I have learned that cleaning the surface of things is not the solution. I need to be with all these feelings, all these eddies of emotion that pull me down. This is reality, my new reality—accepting these feelings, feelings that some might say—that I used to say—were ridiculous. Getting to know them, letting them be until they are ready to move on. Then by expressing them, I honor them as messages from my depths.

I balance my book on top of a of teetering stack of books, roll my chair back, stand up, and offer a silent thank you. Then I turn, head to the dining room and join Wendell for our evening meal.

Acknowledgments

Freud wrote to Jung that psychoanalysis is in essence a cure through love. I would not only agree to this but add that the process of writing a memoir is akin to this; I have felt so much love from the people who have been with me throughout this effort.

My editor, Mary Nilsen, owner of Zion Publishing, believed there was something important in my words and experience that people needed to hear. Her belief in me and this project has been unwavering. She took time to teach me how to make my book more effective, particularly through the writing of vignettes, which allowed for less reliance on second-hand information. I frequently mused to myself that Mary missed her calling as an analyst as she continued to ask questions that took me deeper into what I had learned in analysis. I can't thank her enough.

Barbara Boyd, my book coach, was the first person to see my "shitty first drafts." I felt from the very beginning of our work together that she "got me" and knew what I wanted this memoir to be. Her support and ability to see how my material could be shaped into a memoir was essential for me to keep writing.

Ann Outka, my friend with a huge heart and lawyerly mind, not only pointed out all the missing commas and dashes, but she combed through the chapters several times, each time leaving questions and requests for more information. I learned that lawyers don't look at words in the same way as therapists do. Every time I tackled one of her 'what does this mean?' inquiries, the text transformed for the better.

Many people have read this memoir in its various stages and offered feedback and encouragement. My thanks doesn't seem nearly enough to the following people, but if you knew how helpful your feedback was and how much I appreciated you for being with me on this journey, you would swell with pride: Ruth Foster, Beverly Weismann, Kay Riley, Carol Leech, Nancy Jones, Mason Hiatt, Lisbeth Pelsue, Marcy Mendenhall, Jeanne Williams, Kathi Kuhl, Christine Meinecke, Deborah Hubble.

And of course, my analyst, Denae (not her real name) deserves a great deal of appreciation because her skill as an analyst made all this possible. I will always remember how she asked me if I thought her job was to make me comfortable. It is impossible to put into words how we laughed together at times when I finally got what she had been trying to help me understand. I hope that my rendition of our work together is close to accurate. My thanks to her.

Thanks and acknowledgments are due for any of my former clients who pick up this memoir to peek behind the scenes of my life and discover that we are not that different. That we are all learning to be aware and to be kind.

And speaking of kindness, thanks to the staff at Little Dog Tech for helping me with so many technical difficulties. Your staff, especially Ed, was patient with me when I had no idea what I was asking, let alone what I was doing.

Special thanks to Jenene Armstrong, my personal trainer and health coach, who introduced me to TRX and helped make it possible to exercise regularly even when I was in the throes of furiously writing this memoir. Her commonsense approach to life was a welcome relief to my all-or-nothing thinking, which at times led me to set impossible goals for eating and exercise.

Sarah George, my good friend, stopped by nearly every week when I was writing this memoir to cook for us, act as our seamstress, organize our kitchen, and instruct me on the intricacies of using Word. Sarah is cheerful, creative, real, and compassionate and I would not like to be without her.

Dan Blank, creator of Mastermind and owner of WeGrowMedia, helped me tease out themes of my memoir, assisted me in developing strategies to network with other writers, and helped plan my book launch. Our weekly phone consultations were invaluable.

When I have read acknowledgments in the past in which married authors thanked their partners and said they couldn't have completed their work without their support, I didn't realize how much they likely meant it. Wendell cheered me on when I complained about how hard writing was by saying, "If it was easy, everyone would do it." And he was always available to give me a much-needed hug. Thank you for everything, Wendell.

About the Author

Nicola Mendenhall, known to her family and friends as Nicky, is a retired psychotherapist captivated by the discipline and practice of psychoanalysis. Freudian analysis is, in essence, a cure through love, though she readily admits she was unfamiliar and uncomfortable receiving the psychoanalytic type of love she was offered. Shocked during her sessions, when the analyst's questions brought out her worst qualities, Nicola turned to Freud's analytical attitude. His writings encouraged her to explore the unconscious (a metaphor for all we keep hidden) and to continue her quest to live with greater depth and intimacy, joy and meaning.

Now in her mid-seventies, she remembers fondly her early sixties when she reunited with and married her high school sweetheart, Wendell. Purchasing a home adjacent to a nature trail, they made a joint commitment to staying fit. Nicky is blessed with three sons and two daughters-in-law, and through her marriage she gained two daughters and their husbands. Altogether she and Wendell have six grandchildren.

To contact Nicky:

NickyMendenhall.com
nicola.mendenhall@gmail.com

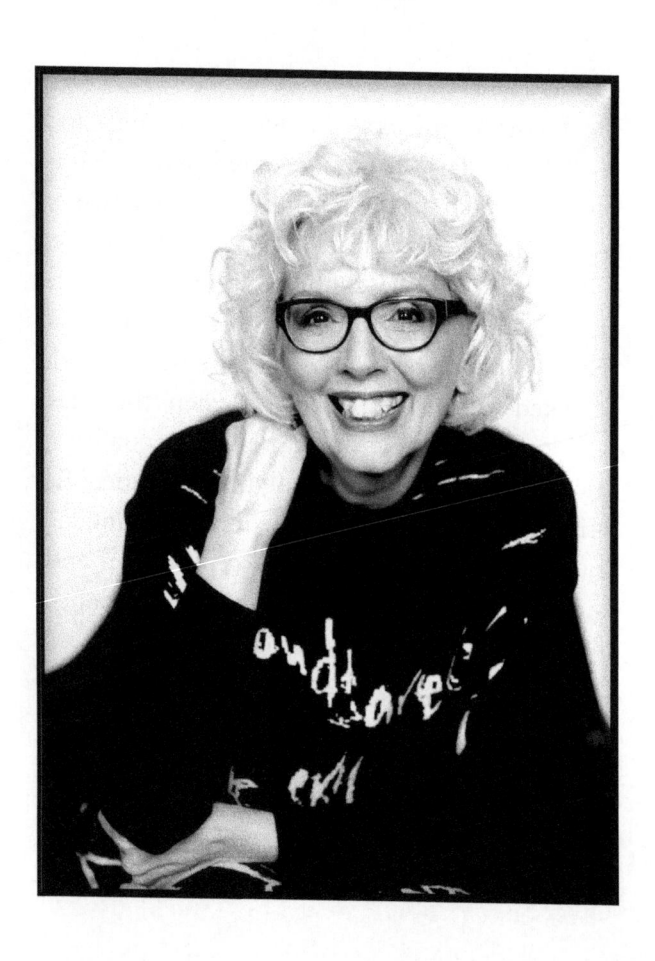

BIBLIOGRAPHY

Aisenstein, M. and de Aisemberg, E.R. (Eds.) (2010). *Psychosomatics Today: A Psychoanalytic Perspective.* London: Karnac Books Ltd.

Anderson, J. (2004). *A Walk on the Beach.* New York: Broadway Books.

Beck, M. (2005). *Leaving the Saints.* New York: Crown Publishers.

Chernin, K. (1995). *A Different Kind of Listening.* New York: HarperCollins Books.

Dinnage, R. (1988). *One to One: Experiences of Psychotherapy.* London: Penguin Books.

Epstein, M. (2001). *Going On Being: Buddhism and the Way of Change.* New York: Broadway Books.

Fingarette, H. (1963). *The Self in Transformation.* New York, London: Basic Books, Inc., Publishers.

Freud, S. (2013). *Psychical (or Mental) Treatment.* Redditch Worcestershire: Read Books Ltd.

Gilbert, E. (2006). *eat, pray, love.* New York: Penguin Group.

Glaser, A. (2005). *A Call to Compassion: Bringing Buddhist Practices of the Heart into the Soul of Psychology.* Berwick, ME: Nicolas-Hays, Inc.

Green, A. (2005). *Key Ideas for a Contemporary Psychoanalysis: Misrecognition and Recognition of the Unconscious.* London: Routledge.

Lindner, R. (1982). *The Fifty-Minute Hour.* New York: MJF Books.

Little, M. I. (1990). *Psychotic Anxieties and Containment.* Northvale, NJ: Jason Aronson.

Mitchell, S. A. (1995). *Freud and Beyond.* New York: Basic Books.

Mitchell, S. A. (2016). *Freud and Beyond.* New York: Basic Books.

Ragen, T. (2009). *The Consulting Room and Beyond.* New York: Routledge.

Seulin, C. S. (Ed.). (2012). *On Freud's "On Beginning the Treatment".* London: Karnac Books Ltd.

Snell, R. (2013). *Uncertainties, Mysteries, Doubts.* New York: Routledge.

van der Kolk, B. A. (2014). *The Body Keeps the Score.* New York: Penguin Group.

Recommended Books

Achterberg, J. (1998). *Uncommon Bonds.* ReVision, 4-10.

Ackerman, D. (2002). *Origami Bridges.* New York: HarperCollins.

Anzieu, D. (1990). *A Skin For Thought.* London: Karnac Books.

Bion, W. R. (1961). *Experiences in Groups and Other Papers.* London: Routledge.

Breger, L. (2000). *Freud: Darkness in the Midst of Vision.* New York: John Wiley & Sons, Inc.

Campbell, J. (2004). *Pathways to Bliss.* Novato, CA: New World Library.

Carotenuto, A. (1981). *The Vertical Labyrinth.* Toronto: Inner City Books.

Cozolino, L. (2010). *The Neuroscience of Psychotherapy* (2nd ed.). New York: W. W. Norton & Company, Inc.

Doyle, B. (2019). *One Long River of Song.* New York: Little, Brown, and Company.

Feldman, M. (2009). *Doubt, Conviction and the Analytic Process.* (B. Joseph, Ed.) London and New York: Routledge.

Fenichel, O. (1945). *The Psychoanalytic Theory of Neurosis.* New York: W. W. Norton & Company

Inc.

Firman, J., & Gila, A. (2010). *A Psychotherapy of Love.* Albany: State University of New York Press.

Forrester, S. (2017). *The Aware Athlete.* La Pine, OR: Earth Lodge Publishing.

Frank, A. W. (2002). *At the Will of the Body.* Boston, New York: Houghton Mifflin Company.

Freud, A. (1966). *The Ego and the Mechanisms of Defense* (2nd ed.). New York: International Universities Press, Inc.

Freud, S. (1966). *Introductory Lectures on Psycho-Analysis.* (J. Strachey, Trans.) New York: W. W. Norton & Company.

Freud, S. (2005). *The Unconscious.* London: Penguin Classics.

Friedman, S. S. (Ed.). (2002). *Analyzing Freud.* New York: New Directions Books.

Grosz, S. (2013). *The Examined Life.* New York: Norton and Co. Inc.

H.D. (1956). *Tribute to Freud.* New York: New Directions.

Hammid, M. (2017). *East West.* New York: Riverhead Books.

Hanna, T. (1970). *Bodies In Revolt.* New York: Dell Publishing Co., Inc.

Hanna, T. (1988). *Somatics.* Reading, MA: Addison-Wesley Publishing Company, Inc.

Herman, N. (1988). *My Kleinian Home.* London:

Free Association Books.

Hunter, V. (1994). *Psychoanalysts Talk*. New York: Guilford Press.

Jennings, P. (2010). *Mixing Minds*. Boston: Wisdom Publications.

Jennings, P. (2017). *To Heal a Wounded Heart*. Boulder: Shamhala.

Langer, S. K. (1957). *Philosophy in a New Key*. Cambridge, MA: Harvard University Press.

Levine, S. S. (1996). *Useful Servants*. Northvale, New Jersey: Jason Aronson Inc.

Lewin, B. D. (1961). *The Psychoanalysis of Elation*. Amazon.

Livingston, S. (2019). *The Virgin of Prince Street*. Lincoln: University of Nebraska Press.

Luepnitz, D. A. (2002). *Schopenhauer's Porcupines*. New York: Basic Books.

Mate, G. (2003). *When the Body Says No*. Hoboken, N. J.: John Wiley & Sons, Inc.

Milner, M. (2010). *The Hands of the Living God*. Hove: Routledge.

Mitchell, S. A. (1995). *Freud and Beyond*. New York: Basic Books.

Molino, A. (Ed.). (1997). *Freely Associated*. New York, New York: Free Association Books Ltd.

Oakes, M. (1987). *The Stone Speaks*. Wilmette, Illinois: Chiron Publications.

Obama, M. (2018). *Becoming*. New York: Crown Publishing Group.

Ogden, T. H. (1989). *The Primitive Edge Of Experience*. Northvale, New Jersey: Jason Aronson Inc.

Ogden, T. H. (2009). *Rediscovering Psychoanalysis*. Hove: Routledge, England.

Orbach, S. (2000). *The Impossibility of Sex*. New York: Scribner.

Parsons, W. B. (1999). *The Enigma of the Oceanic Feeling*. Oxford: Oxford University Press.

Person, E. S., & Fonagy, P. (Eds.). (1995). *On Freud's "Creative Writers and Day-Dreaming."* New Haven: Yale University Press.

Phillips, A. (2014). *Becoming Freud*. New Haven: Yale University Press.

Pines, D. (1993). *A Woman's Unconscious Use of Her Body*. Hove: Routledge.

Roiphe, K. (2016). *The Violet Hour*. New York: The Dial Press.

Rothberg, D., & Masters, R. A. (Eds.). (1998). *ReVision* (Vol. 21). Washington, D.C.: Heldref Publications.

Safran, J. D. (Ed.). (2003). *Psychoanalysis and Buddhism*. Somerville: Wisdom Publications.

Sarno, J. E. (2006). *The Divided Mind*. New York: Harper.

Schafer, R. (1983). *The Analytic Attitude*. New York: Basic Books, Inc.

Severino, S. K. (2009). *Becoming Fire*. New York: Monkfish Book Publishing Company.

Shinder, J. (Ed.). (2000). *Tales from the Couch*.

New York, New York: William Morrow.

Stein, M. M. (2007). *The Lonely Patient.* New York: Harper Perennial.

Suzuki, D. T.; Fromm, Erich; De Martino, Richard. (1963). *Zen Buddhism and Psychoanalysis.* New York: Grove Press, Inc.

Tiberghien, S. M. (2007). *Looking for Gold.* Einsiedeln: Daimon.

Ulanov, A. B. (2001). *Attacked by Poison Ivy.* York Beach, NY: Nicolas-Hays, Inc.

Ulrich, D. (2018). *Zen Camera.* New York: Watson-Guptill.

Vaughan, F. (1985). *The Inward Arc.* Boston: New Science Library.

Vaughan, F. (2005). *Shadows of the Sacred.* Lincoln, NE: An Authors Guild Backinprint.com Edition.

Wheelis, J. (2019). *the known, the secret, the forgotten.* New York: W. W. Norton & Company.

Wolff-Salin, M. (1988). *No Other Light.* New York: Crossroad Publishing Company.

Young-Eisendrath, P., & Miller, M. E. (Eds.). (2000). *The Psychology of Mature Spirituality.* London: Routledge.

CPSIA information can be obtained
at www.ICGtesting.com
Printed in the USA
LVHW080947080222
710548LV00018B/634

9 781735 795867